## Praise for Dr. Aric A. Prather and *The Seven-Day Sleep Prescription*

"The vastly knowledgeable and genuinely brilliant Dr. Aric Prather can take detailed scientific concepts and distill them into wondrous bite-size chunks, digestible to all. An easy yet most effective how-to guide on sleep."
—Dr. Matthew Walker, *New York Times* bestselling author of *Why We Sleep* and director of the Center for Human Sleep Science, University of California, Berkeley

"Deceptively simple and refreshingly straightforward, *The Seven-Day Sleep Prescription* is an immediately useful guide to getting better sleep. Aric Prather is an internationally-recognized scientific authority on sleep health and his advice can help just about anyone sleep more restfully in just a week."
—Dr. Michael Grandner, director of the Sleep and Health Research Program, University of Arizona College of Medicine

"*The Seven-Day Sleep Prescription* is a practical guide to improving your sleep and enhancing your life. Prather offers a set of transformative and doable changes in sleep habits that can make you healthier, happier, and more productive."
—Tom Boyce, MD, author of *The Orchid and the Dandelion*

"*The Seven-Day Sleep Prescription* is a game changer. It's an original and effective take on how we sleep and why so many of us struggle to do it well. A must-have for anyone looking to improve their waking life by fixing their sleeping one."
—Dr. Sara Mednick, author of *The Power of the Downstate* and *Take a Nap! Change Your Life*.

"Through a series of seven sensible steps, Dr. Prather guides us to relearn what our bodies and brains already know: we can use our voluntary, waking behaviors to influence the involuntary, restorative process of sleep."
—Dr. Daniel Buysse, director of the Center for Sleep and Circadian Science, University of Pittsburgh School of Medicine

PENGUIN LIFE

# THE SEVEN-DAY SLEEP PRESCRIPTION

Aric A. Prather, PhD, is a professor of psychiatry and behavioral sciences at the University of California, San Francisco, where he codirects the Aging, Metabolism, and Emotions Center. He is also a licensed clinical psychologist who helps lead the UCSF Insomnia Clinic where he practices cognitive behavioral therapy to treat patients with insomnia. He directs a robust research program focused on the causes and consequences of insufficient sleep, which has been continuously funded by the National Institutes of Health. A self-proclaimed sleep evangelist, Dr. Prather has dedicated his career to raising awareness about the importance of sleep health, and to advocate for sleep opportunity as a basic human right.

# THE SEVEN-DAY SLEEP PRESCRIPTION

## Seven Days to Unlocking Your Best Rest

ARIC A. PRATHER, PhD

PENGUIN LIFE

AN IMPRINT OF

PENGUIN BOOKS

PENGUIN LIFE

UK | USA | Canada | Ireland | Australia
India | New Zealand | South Africa

Penguin Life is part of the Penguin Random House group of companies
whose addresses can be found at global.penguinrandomhouse.com.

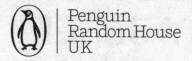

First published in the United States of America by Penguin Life, Penguin Books,
an imprint of Penguin Random House LLC 2022
First published in Great Britain by Penguin Life 2022

002

Book design by Daniel Lagin
Printed and bound in Great Britain by Clays Ltd, Elcograf S.p.A.

The authorized representative in the EEA is Penguin Random House Ireland,
Morrison Chambers, 32 Nassau Street, Dublin D02 YH68

A CIP catalogue record for this book is available from the British Library

ISBN: 978-0-241-60034-4

www.greenpenguin.co.uk

Penguin Random House is committed to a
sustainable future for our business, our readers
and our planet. This book is made from Forest
Stewardship Council® certified paper.

*This book is dedicated to my wife, Michelle, and my two boys, Spencer and Jackson. You may disturb my sleep at times, but you also give me the confidence to dream.*

# CONTENTS

# INTRODUCTION

## YOU WERE BUILT TO SLEEP

A FEW YEARS AGO, JUST AFTER MY YOUNGER SON WAS BORN, I SPENT a long night holding him as he slept on my chest. He was just a couple weeks old, still so small he could fit inside my two palms. Like any new parent in that situation, I was exhausted—my eyes felt sandy, and I could barely keep them open. Meanwhile, he was deeply asleep, his slow, rhythmic baby breath whooshing in my ear. I knew though that the minute I tried to slowly (excruciatingly slowly!) lay him down, he'd pop awake and start shrieking in protest. So I muscled my eyes open and held him a little longer. As a sleep scientist, I knew what sleep was doing for him and for his little developing brain: Consolidating memories. Building new neural synapses. Washing away the byproducts of daytime brain processes with a cleansing flush of cerebrospinal fluid. Lowering his blood pressure to relax his little nervous system. Releasing human growth hormone throughout the body, which promotes healing, regeneration, and growth.

It wasn't the first night I'd spent holding a kid through the wee hours when all I wanted was to be asleep myself, and it wouldn't be the last. But that night I found myself thinking a lot about how much *work* sleep can be. In our sleep clinic at the University of California, San Francisco (UCSF), we have (metaphorically, at least) a line out the door of people needing help with their sleep. For many, sleep is tricky and elusive—it's a source of stress and anxiety, rather than relaxation and restoration. For some, it feels like a "skill" they never quite had a grasp on, a lifetime of being a "bad sleeper." For others, it's a skill that has vanished suddenly, with no explanation—where did it go?

Like eating, drinking, and breathing, we need to sleep to survive. If we stopped sleeping, we would die. Sure, it would take a while, but sleep is just as much an essential, life-supporting process as those other things—like food, water, and oxygen. Eventually, without it, our bodies begin to shut down. So why on earth can something that should be so natural, instinctual, and automatic be so hard?

I study sleep for a living, and I'll tell you right off the bat that there's usually one major thing that gets in the way of sleep: *you*.

I don't mean just you. I mean all of us. We're *great* at getting in the way of our own sleep. We don't mean to. And we're not making obviously bad choices. In the sleep clinic, my colleagues and I treat hundreds of patients per year who are struggling to achieve good sleep. By the time they come to us, they've tried everything. They've done the usual sleep hygiene stuff, like making their sleeping space calming and dark and cool. They've tried medications. They've often been referred by doctors or therapists. For many, sleep has become so loaded with difficulty that *anxiety* about whether or not they'll be able to sleep tonight is the thing that keeps them from sleeping—ironic, yes, but also a very powerful and a hard to break anti-sleep cycle.

A big part of our problem is that we aren't living in a world that's set up to allow us to sleep well. For many, sleep comes last. There are so many other pressures and priorities. We make the best decisions we can throughout the day: To get our work done. To succeed and achieve. To pay the bills. To support our kids and partners. But so many of those decisions—which make plenty of sense *in the moment*—catch up to us at the end of the day. Because of these seemingly small choices, we end up with dysregulated circadian rhythms, or not enough oomph in our homeostatic sleep drive. We close our eyes with sleep-hormone-blocking stimulants like caffeine still permeating our whole system, because we didn't calculate the half-life of that last cup of tea, or soda, or coffee. We sabotage our deep, restorative slow-wave sleep—which we need to clean the metabolic gunk out of the brain after another long day. Our comfy beds become, surprisingly, a trigger for wakefulness rather than sleepiness, a problem that's compounded the longer we struggle with sleep without knowing how to break the "conditioned arousal" we are training in our brains and bodies.

Sleep isn't something we *do* as much as it is something that happens *to* us. A lot of it is about letting go, getting out of our own way, and training our bodies to recognize the cues at night, and *throughout the day*, that tell it what it should be doing, and when. The decisions you make that shape your sleep don't start when you lie down at night. They start the minute you open your eyes in the morning.

Most people who struggle with sleep don't need to be told how urgent sleep is for their health—they already know. They need to be given a simple map of how to live their days in a way that sets them up for great sleep *tonight*.

## Sleep: The Glue That Holds Your Life Together

Most of us never wonder how sleep works until it stops working. I didn't think much about sleep (other than the fact that I could have used more of it) until I was in graduate school, training as a clinical-health psychologist, studying how psychological and behavioral factors, like stress and sleep, impact the immune system. Originally, my work focused on identifying factors that predict how people respond to vaccines. Vaccinations are critical in the prevention of disease, and while they are on the whole effective, we don't all mount the same level of protection to the same vaccine. I wanted to understand how things like mood, stress, sleep, and other factors predicted people's immune response, in this case to a hepatitis B vaccination. The more research I did, the more one thing became crystal clear: *Insufficient sleep affected the kind of response people had to the vaccination*. People who got less sleep were less able to build the antibodies that would protect against hep B.[1]

We've since found the same is true for people who get the flu vaccine.[2] Even more astounding, when we brought people into the lab and shot a live cold virus into their nose, people who typically get fewer than six hours of sleep per night were *four times more likely* to develop a cold than those who usually sleep more than seven hours per night.[3] Everyone in the study had the exact same level of exposure to the cold-causing virus—but they had vastly different immune responses. Sleep was the factor that somehow conferred a strong level of protection.

There's a lot about our lives and our health we can't control. But sleep is one of the areas where we can see a huge transformation with a few concrete changes. It turns out that improving our sleep can lead to improvements in many other aspects of our life, including how we feel, what we eat, how we learn, and how we react to others during the day, things that are often harder for us to change on our own. When we sleep better we feel better, we're more creative and engaged, have more energy to exercise, and have a greater tendency to pile our plates with healthy foods and colorful fruits and veggies. When you sleep better, your whole life improves, creating a foundation for health and well-being. As one former patient told me, "You gave me my sleep back, and it changed my life."

Today, I spend most of my time at UCSF, carrying out clinical research to better understand how and why sleep is so critical for health. I have the privilege of serving as a clinician in our UCSF insomnia clinic, where we implement cognitive behavioral therapy for insomnia (CBTI), which comprises a set of empirically validated treatments to promote long-lasting restorative sleep. I've treated hundreds of people desperate for a good night's sleep—a few of their stories appear in this book—and my enchantment with sleep has only grown stronger. While each person's specific sleep challenge and cure are unique, a major theme runs through my work. For most of us who have trouble sleeping, the root of the problem can usually be traced to behaviors and decisions that make sense in the short term, but end up undermining how sleep works naturally.

Mark is a great example. He suddenly developed insomnia when his son was diagnosed with autism spectrum disorder. During the overwhelming period when he and his wife were trying to wrap their heads around the diagnosis and seek out services for their son, Mark couldn't relax his mind enough to sleep. He started going to bed earlier, trying to give himself the best opportunity for sleep, but just lay awake tossing and turning. After a bad night, he'd sleep in late or nap during the day, trying to get as much shut-eye as possible. But that just made it even harder for him to fall asleep at night. His schedule became disjointed, his body confused about when he needed to rest or be alert. And his anxiety increased, because now on top of his acute stress—concern for his son and getting the best interventions—he was chronically sleep-deprived and chronically stressed about not getting enough rest.

Anyone worried about a high-stakes exam or a crumbling relationship or ailing loved one would probably agree that when you're stressed out, you don't sleep as well. And anyone up all night with a baby, a deadline, a nightmare, or a bout of anxiety knows that when we don't sleep well, we're more sensitive to stress during the day. Little problems feel like big ones. The point here is that our sleep and mood and levels of daily stress all influence one another. Targeting one piece of the cycle automatically helps the other two. So if we improve our sleep, we also give ourselves a greater chance of feeling better and having the coping resources to deal with the slings and arrows of the day. And the better we feel and the more coping resources we have during the day, the better we are able to drift off to sleep.

But it isn't just stress or worry that gets in the way of sleep. Sometimes sleep is related to other physical or mental health conditions. When one patient started treatment at our clinic, her chronic back pain was keeping her up much of the night. Pain stopped her from sleeping; fragmented and interrupted sleep made the pain worse. When we get less sleep, it decreases our pain threshold.[4] Sleep can't erase pain completely—but it can turn down the volume. And being better rested improves our physical and mental resources for dealing with pain, which in turn gives us greater confidence in our capacity to heal. For this patient, healthy sleep wasn't just about getting better rest— it was also about enhancing her ability to heal her body, and giving her enough energy and optimism to help her stay mentally healthy as well. When we don't sleep, the world not only feels worse, it looks worse: we have more of a negative filter and fewer cognitive and emotional resources. Even the most minor stressors can throw us for a loop when we are short on sleep.

Sleep often ends up being the last thing on our to-do list. Really, it should be the first. It's an "essential nutrient" that we all need for health, longevity, and vitality, and it's not one we all have equal access to.

## "Sleep Access" Is Not Evenly Distributed

Sometimes sleep has to do with things beyond our own bodies—with social and economic factors and other systemic issues in our environments and communities. Angel, a mother of two young children, revealed during her intake interview that she lived in a dangerous neighborhood. There had been a recent shooting near her home, an occurrence that was becoming more and more common. She'd started staying up all night to watch over her children while they slept. Her insomnia, born of a strong need and desire to protect her children, had snowballed into chronic, heightened vigilance. Her treatment plan involved lowering her hyper-aroused threat response so she could harness the benefits of restorative sleep.

We know now that sufficient and restorative sleep is not evenly distributed across populations—there are clear sleep inequities. For example: on average, African Americans and low-income individuals report shorter, less restorative sleep than people in other racial demographics and higher socioeconomic groups.[5] A large part of my work now involves trying to understand the social processes and determinants that contribute to sleep disparities in the population. Though it's rarely seen this way, sleep is a vital social justice issue. Everyone deserves the right to a restful night's sleep.

While social and policy changes are needed to address sleep and health disparities, for many the capacity for healthy sleep is personal, residing within each of us. No matter how much of a fight sleep has been for you, let's start with some good news:

*you are built to sleep.* Underneath all of the anti-sleep conditioning you're probably battling, your body knows how to do it. What we're going to do in this book is clear away those obstacles so that it remembers how—and so you can get back your sense of "sleep mastery."

This book doesn't replace medical treatment or serve as a public health program. (There are additional resources at the end of the book that can help you determine whether you might want to speak with your doctor, as well as point you toward treatment options and next steps.) What this book does do is follow the innovative premise of our insomnia clinic and many other sleep centers around the world: that better sleep is about harnessing what the body already knows how to do, freeing ourselves from the behaviors that adversely affect sleep, and reinforcing the behaviors that restore us to our natural sleep rhythm.

## Become Your Own Sleep Scientist to Unlock the Secret to Your Sleep

Sleep is universal yet personal. There are some baseline things that are true about sleep for all of us, and of course we'll cover those constants here. But there's no single, all-encompassing model that works for everyone. The key is to find the specific parameters within these core practices that we'll go through, day by day, that work best for *you*.

A lot of us suffer because we're trying to achieve a sleep model that ultimately isn't going to work for us. We align our

sleep habits to others, or to work demands. We don't pay attention to—or even notice—our bodies' unique natural sleep cues
and rhythms. Some of us have unrealistic expectations about
what good sleep looks like. We focus on that one spectacular
night—you know the one. The one where you fell dead asleep
and woke up in that very same position the next morning feeling amazing. That was an exceptional night, indeed, but certainly not the measuring stick to evaluate all your future nights
of sleep.

We all need food and oxygen, but it doesn't mean we eat and
breathe the same. I'm not going to tell you what time to go to
bed, or what time to wake up, or even exactly how many hours
to get (though I will make some strong suggestions based on
what we know the *average* person needs). I'm going to help you
find *your* natural rhythms and leverage them for better sleep.

Your mission for this week, if you choose to accept it, is to
become your own sleep scientist. The information in this book
is broadly applicable—these are the most foundational, essential sleep tools that everybody needs to have. But when it comes
to sleep, we all suffer from *different* challenges. That's why, when
people seek sleep treatments, they are personalized. So, one of
the first things we'll discuss in this book is how to keep a sleep
diary, a simple tool for tracking your sleep patterns across the
next seven days so that we can find solutions based on *your* data.

Some of the techniques we try this week will resonate with
you; others may feel (at least at first) less impactful. That's to be
expected. But also recognize that like most behavior changes,
some of the benefits won't appear overnight, and may take a bit

of practice to master. Each individual practice is one step toward better sleep; however, they tend to work better together. I like to think of this as a kind of "recipe" for sleep. There's some wiggle room for substitutions, but if you leave out a key ingredient, it's probably not going to work. Just like with baking, the chemistry works best when you stick to the recipe and include all the ingredients. If you really give these strategies a try and record the results with the sleep diary I'll provide, you'll begin to figure out what works for you even faster. You get out of this what you put in. You can be a consumer, or you can be a collaborator—and I hope you choose the latter!

Sleep is an amazing medicine. It's so potent, it can help with any number of the ills that plague us. You probably already know that sleep is good for you, and that it feels good to get it. Well, the science is showing us just how true that is. Good sleep boosts the immune system.[6] It regulates metabolism.[7] It makes you happier. It makes you a better, more empathetic partner and a more patient parent.[8] It can improve your productivity and creativity at work and boost your energy so you can actually squeeze in that extra (or first!) workout during the week.[9] It sharpens the mind and can actually clear toxins out of the brain that build up over time, including those thought to play a role in neurodegenerative diseases—I sometimes call sleep "the dishwasher of the brain."[10] But just like a dishwasher, you have to let it run the whole cycle. And as I said, the biggest block to good sleep is often *ourselves*—our daytime behaviors and misguided beliefs about how to sleep that get in the way of the natural restorative process our bodies want so badly to perform.

Here's the bottom line: sleep is natural, but it's not always easy. As a human being, you are biologically built to sleep. *But the obstacles are real.* Digital distractions, stress, the environments where you live and sleep, and even larger systemic issues like race and class put pressures on our biology ... and it bleeds into sleep. Many of us have been steeped in a culture that devalues sleep: ever heard the expression "You can sleep when you're dead"? We all have responsibilities, big goals, big pressures. You're here on this planet for a purpose. But you can't do any of what you really want to do if you can't sleep.

We each have our unique challenges. Maybe your challenge is figuring out how to prioritize sleep when the rest of life encroaches. Or maybe you've been prioritizing it, and still struggling. Maybe your sleep isn't bad, but you're an optimizer, a hacker who wants to maximize the restoration you can get each day. To all of you: this book is for you! No matter your starting point, the strategies here, spread out over the next week, are the tried-and-true tools that we know improve sleep, and in doing so, improve well-being and joy.

So for the next seven days, we're going to tackle one tiny habit per day. Each habit-switch will show you how to clear away the most common obstacles to sleep, and instead create a strong association with sleep cues, unique to you, that will help you lay back and let sleep work its magic. What this book is going to teach you is how to get out of your own way, so that your body can do what it was built to do: *sleep.*

# BEFORE WE BEGIN

## Have You Covered the Basics?

For the purposes of our week together, I'm going to assume that you already know about basic "sleep hygiene"—if you're holding this book, you've probably already tried the basic stuff that's out there. In this book, we're not going to spend a lot of time on how you should keep your room dark and your phone downstairs. Instead, we're going deeper: to the "sleep pressure points" within your biology and your life, and how to engage them to move your sleep in the right direction.

That said, sleep hygiene is talked about a lot for a reason: this stuff is important. You can do everything I suggest over the next seven days, and still sabotage yourself by not practicing the intro-level stuff. So if you're a sleep hygiene expert, this list can serve as a refresher and a double-check to catch any sleep best practices that have lapsed (it happens); if you're new to the idea of sleep hygiene, this will be your Sleep 101 crash course and get you off on the right foot.

## Sleep Basics Checklist

❑ **Is your room dark?** Lights, including blue spectrum light from your tablet and computer screens, TVs, and phones, can interrupt the production of important sleep-inducing chemicals in the brain. Solution: Use blackout curtains or a comfortable eye mask. Limit exposure to screens a few hours before bed (more on this later) or try a blue light filter on your device to dampen down exposure.

❑ **Is your room cool?** One of the things that has to happen for sleep to come is for your core body temperature to drop. It's a key part of falling asleep. If possible, lower the temp a bit in your sleeping area. The sweet spot seems to be a room temperature of 65°F (18.3°C), though there is some wiggle room based on your own preferences (range of 60°F to 67°F). Solution: Drop the heat (or turn up the AC) and add a blanket. Dark and cool is what you're going for.

❑ **Is your bedroom clutter- and distraction-free?** Eliminate work clutter and other stuff that might cause you any anxiety or feelings of "I need to get that done." This is an "out of sight, out of mind" situation. Solution: Stash your laptop someplace else. Pack away work papers. Stuff that unfolded pile of laundry in the closet. When you sit in bed and look around your room, it should calm you, not activate you. Life has a lot of clutter—try to keep it in another room if you can.

❑ **Is your phone attached to your hand?** No judgment—mine usually is. But I do try to follow the advice of my fellow sleep experts and not *sleep* with it literally in my hand. We'll be talking more about phones, blue light, and when you need to worry about devices disrupting your sleep later, but for now, just know that a phone next to your head at night is generally not the best for sleep, especially if sleep is something that's been eluding you. Solution: Leave your phone in another room at bedtime. Or, if that's not possible (many people don't have any other way to set an alarm, for instance) plug it in on the other side of the room, or in a nearby hallway or bathroom—just get it out of your sleep space.

❏ **Do you know your sleep data?** A lot of us use wearables and apps to track our sleep. I study sleep for a living, so you can be sure that I have a closet full of devices designed to track every conceivable aspect of sleep. These can be powerful tools to illuminate sleep behavior, but they can also quickly become a source of angst. So often I meet with a patient who's distraught that their wrist-worn device, a sleep oracle of sorts, records a night of 0 percent deep sleep. It's unlikely that the device is accurate, but the distress it causes is 100 percent real. A couple of years ago, sleep researchers coined the phrase "orthosomnia" to refer to the specific type of insomnia brought on by sleep-measurement devices.[1] Solution: For this week as you work your way through this book (and in my opinion, for the rest of your life after that!), don't get too wrapped up in the sleep data from these devices if you use them. Instead, I'd like to ask you to rely on a sleep diary that you'll use to track your sleep patterns yourself. Technology has come a long way when it comes to sleep measurement, and the future is bright. But let's try the old-school sleep diary approach for this week.

## Start Your Sleep Diary . . . Right Now

If you were to come into my sleep clinic, this is the first thing I'd have you do. In fact, we'd do it before we even started working on your sleep. The data from people's sleep diary are extraordinarily valuable—it's how we figure out how to tailor our interventions to help them most effectively. They come in, we talk about their problem, and then I send them away with a sleep diary and instructions to come back in a week.

Our timeline here is compressed, and I can't burst off the pages of this book and customize a plan for you. But that's exactly what I'm going to ask *you* to do over the next seven days: customize your sleep plan. Each day is going to offer a tried-and-true intervention that, honestly, we do with just about everyone who comes in. Meanwhile, I'm going to ask you to keep this diary every day. And at the end of the week, we're going to analyze your data and get even more granular about how *you* specifically can tailor your sleep methodologies to be better for you.

Don't rely on a wearable for this. I want you to do this handwritten sleep diary, even if you do wear something that tracks sleep. Relying on devices and apps usually means we miss part of the larger picture—when *you* are the one tracking instead of an AI, you can see patterns in your behavior that would otherwise be lost or obscured. And the process of keeping a sleep diary in and of itself can be very therapeutic. Sleep diaries themselves are one of our well-researched interventions. So we're going to start yours as soon as you start day one. If you flip quickly to the back of this book, you'll find a section with several blank sleep diary templates, ready for you to use. Feel free to write directly in the book—but I also recommend making copies of one of the blank templates before you start filling it in, so you can keep this practice up beyond these next seven days. I do want you to use the template: at the end of this week, we're going to be doing some calculations to evaluate your sleep data, and that's easiest to do in the format provided!

Feel free to start your sleep diary immediately—or after you start day one of your week of being a sleep scientist.

# SET YOUR (INTERNAL) CLOCK

LET'S COMPARE HUMANS TO SOME OF OUR FELLOW COMPANIONS ON this Earth. Giraffes sleep for less than five hours across the twenty-four-hour day, while lions spend an amazing sixteen to twenty hours resting or sleeping over that same period. The albatross, an enormous airplane of a bird that can travel ten thousand miles in a single journey, can achieve REM sleep *while in flight*. And hippos? They sleep underwater, unconsciously surfacing while sleeping in order to breathe. Even flowers have an internal clock, coded into their cells, that tells them when to open and close. For as many types of organisms as there are out there, there are types of sleep rhythms.

We humans are fairly boring sleepers—most adults need a minimum of seven hours of sleep per night,[1] and we can't even swim while we're doing it. And perhaps more so than hippos and flowers, we struggle with sleep. A big reason? Our natural sleep cycles are out of whack.

Once upon a time, human sleep cycles were yoked more

firmly to the natural world—we woke with the morning light and wound down into sleep as the sun disappeared. Then we discovered fire, and everything went downhill from there. Now we have electricity. Technology. Schedules that are not so much governed by the natural world but by the new digital one we've created. We have emails to return, Netflix to watch, passions to pursue. We're no longer hunter-gatherers who wake and sleep with the sun—we have jobs that get us up early and keep us up late. We're awash in artificial light beaming at us from light-bulbs, phones, and laptop screens long after our distant ancestors would have been deep into their sleep cycles. If our natural biological rhythms were allowed to be the boss of us, maybe falling asleep and waking up would be as effortless for us as it is for the flower.

Is the answer to go off the grid, live in the woods, and sleep and wake with the sun again like our ancient ancestors? Maybe! A really creative research study found that participants who went camping in the Colorado wilderness for a weekend and weren't allowed to use artificial lighting at night (no flashlights, headlamps, nothing) showed a 69 percent shift in their biological sleep/wake rhythm compared to those who stayed home.[2] But my guess is that most people—even those who have sleep struggles—are probably not willing to cut ties with the civilized world completely in order to fix them. We need to figure out a way—within this electrical, digital, twenty-four-hour, inter-connected, fast-paced modern world—to stabilize and re-sync our sleep drivers so that we can get the kind of deep restorative sleep we still need as humans.

That's why we're going to start this project of fixing your sleep first thing in the morning. When people have trouble sleeping, a lot of attention gets paid to bedtime. But setting yourself up for successful sleep doesn't start at bedtime, or an hour before bedtime, or whenever you start to wind down for the night. It starts the minute you wake up.

## When Do You Wake Up?

Five a.m.? Seven? Noon?

If you're expecting a lecture about the early bird getting the worm, it's not going to come from me. I work with lots of people each year in our sleep clinic at UCSF, working on individualized solutions for their insomnia and other sleep difficulties. And I've rarely told anyone they needed to get up early, or really at any particular time. I don't care what time you wake up. I only care that you wake up at the *same time* every day.

My youngest son is five years old. I mention that to make clear that I have a natural, unstoppable alarm clock built into my life—even on the laziest of weekends, I couldn't sleep in if I tried. But even if I didn't have this kiddo appearing at my bedside at six o'clock sharp, wanting pancakes and to discuss [insert Marvel Avenger], I still wouldn't try to sleep in on the weekends—not anymore. The luxurious sleepy Sundays of my pre-parenting life are far in the rear-view mirror, and it's because of the data.

If you're like most people (and me, before the science of sleep became my career), you spend your work week running a little short on sleep, then you try to "catch up" on the weekends (or whenever your days off roll around) by tacking on an extra hour or two. This sleep debt that builds up across the week is called "social jet lag." Teenagers are the most striking example of this. There are no teens in my home yet (thank goodness) but I certainly remember being one. Beyond the mood swings and the angst, I remember sleeping in—a lot. Teenagers often experience a shift in their sleep rhythm known as "delayed sleep phase" that increases their biological preference to go to bed later at night and wake up later in the morning. Meanwhile, schools start early—much earlier than teens biologically want to awaken—and it produces *sleep debt* across the week that compounds into sleeping in on the weekend. "Catching up" on sleep like this makes logical sense: If you're thirsty, drink more water. If you're tired, give your body more sleep. Unfortunately though, for someone struggling with sleep, this strategy often backfires. It not only doesn't work, it can actively work against you.

Your body loves to anticipate your next action or need. It makes insulin in anticipation of a meal, and melatonin in anticipation of sleep. It knows to do these things because of cues in your routine and environment—cues that start the moment you open your eyes, and which accumulate through the day. If your routine is erratic, your body gets confused about what it needs to be doing and how it should be using its resources. No, you don't have to become an automaton doing the same thing every day, eating the same meals, etc.! But figuring out a consistent wake-up time is the *number one thing* I do with people who come into the sleep clinic. And that's because it's the most powerful regulator of the two natural internal processes that cause sleep.

## What Makes Us Sleep?

You have two main "drivers" of sleep: your *homeostatic sleep drive* and your *circadian rhythm*. These two natural, internal processes in your body work together (though they are independent) to keep you awake when you need to be awake, and asleep when you need to be asleep. They also need to be in sync for you to get great sleep. When they become dysregulated, you start to run into trouble.

Your homeostatic sleep drive is essentially "pressure" for sleep that builds up the longer you're awake. Picture a balloon. It's flat and empty the moment you open your eyes in the morning. As you go through your day, it gradually begins to inflate, filling up with sleepiness. When it's at this optimal amount—picture a perfectly inflated balloon—you feel the need for sleep. Your eyes get heavy, you climb into bed, and drift off. When you take a nap, you're basically "letting some of the air" out of the balloon, or relieving some of that sleep pressure.

What causes sleep pressure to increase? Well honestly, we aren't 100 percent sure—as much as we've mapped the human brain during sleep, there's still a lot we don't know about sleep even though it's one of the most basic and essential biological processes of the human experience. But one of the leading hypotheses is that our sleep drive is hooked to the buildup of certain neurochemicals—which are byproducts of brain activity. A specific neurochemical responsible for sleepiness is, we think, *adenosine*. If you've ever taken a science class, you might remember learning about ATP, or *adenosine triphosphate,* the energy source for all the living cells in our body. While you're awake, adenosine builds up in the brain. As you sleep, that neurochemical drains away. Caffeine, one of the most common ways to keep ourselves awake despite an ever-growing sleep balloon, works because it engages in a biochemical battle with adenosine in the brain. There's basically a fight between the two molecules that breaks out in your brain, and caffeine blocks adenosine uptake by brain receptors. It works really effectively for a while, but when it wears off, you can have a sudden crash of exhaustion as that sleep pressure rebounds right back.

So that's the first important piece: you wake up, that balloon starts to inflate, and once that sleep pressure reaches its optimal level, your body wants to fall asleep. But your homeostatic sleep drive isn't the only thing regulating your sleep cycle. If it were, you might just drop off throughout the day and night whenever that balloon filled up, even if that happened to be in the middle of a meeting or while you were driving. Which brings us to the *circadian rhythm.*

Your circadian rhythm is, most basically, your "master clock" that governs the rhythm of all your body's processes—including sleep and wakefulness. All of the cells in your body, all of your organs, including your brain, have rhythms. There's an ebb and flow of processes and activity throughout the course of a twenty-four-hour day. That master clock that controls all of this lives deep in an area of the brain called the suprachiasmatic nucleus, or SCN, which is found in the hypothalamus, a small but influential area of the brain that controls everything from the release of hormones, to thirst, to body temperature, and more. It also determines your "alertness rhythm" throughout the day. In general, our alertness tends to spike higher in the morning, dip in the afternoon, rebound slightly, and then wane slowly through the evening until we need to go to sleep.

So how does this "master clock" decide how to regulate us? In two main ways.

The first is *internal*—your master clock's rhythms are shaped by your genes and the proteins they produce. This is something you don't have much control over. It's written in your DNA. Like a lot of other traits (your hair color, your preference for sweet versus salty, whether you can roll your tongue or not) you inherited a circadian preference from your parents and ancestors. You probably already know whether you're a morning or night person by nature. You can certainly push against your genetic circadian preference, but some people find that more challenging than others. It may always be hard for you to stay up late; or you may manage to shift your wake time earlier because of a job schedule or simply because you want to seize the day, but may always feel sluggish or foggy for a while, like you're fighting your body's preprogrammed settings. That's because, well, you are. (This isn't to discourage you or imply that it's a losing battle—just to realize that there's nothing wrong with you if you do have trouble moving your bed or wake times.)

The second category of factors that influence your circadian rhythm are *external*. The "arousal systems" in your brain are, at all times, gathering information from your surroundings. *Darkness* is a huge trigger for sleepiness. First, photoreceptors within the retina sense light or the lack thereof. That information travels through neural pathways in the brain to the hypothalamus, the walnut-sized control center of your nervous system, which notes the waning of the day and pings the pineal gland to begin releasing melatonin, the sleepiness-inducing hormone that's been pilled and bottled and put on shelves all over grocery stores and pharmacies to help the sleep-challenged make it to dreamland. It works in reverse, too: when you're exposed to light (especially direct sunlight), the opposite happens—melatonin release is suppressed.

The external cues that influence circadian rhythm are not limited to daylight—though that's a strong one. There are all kinds of "landmarks" throughout your day that give unconscious yet powerful signals to your brain about where exactly you are in your twenty-four-hour cycle, which allows your body to optimize and prepare for what's next, a process called *entrainment*. We call these powerful environmental cues *zeitgebers*, German for "time-givers." The term refers to anything in the environment or routine of a living organism that has the power to change its internal timekeeping clock—in other words, its circadian rhythm. These zeitgebers have the most power over us: Daylight, or the waning of it. When we eat. When we exercise. Temperature. Even social interactions. These elements of your environment or routine become something your body not just responds to, but *anticipates*. It does this to optimize, to maximize your biological efficiency.

Because of these zeitgebers, your body will produce cortisol in anticipation of you waking up—before your alarm clock even goes off. That way, when your alarm does go off, your energy is already rising; you're ready to wake. It will produce insulin in anticipation of glucose flooding your system during a meal—before you're anywhere near sitting down with your knife and fork. By the time you're chewing and swallowing your food, your metabolic systems are ready to process it into energy and nutrients. And in response to the waning light and dropping temperature of evening, along with other cues in your evening routine, your body will begin releasing melatonin ahead of bedtime, readying your system for slumber.

To sum up: our circadian rhythms are the product of a swirl of factors. They are partially genetically predetermined, partially shaped by our immediate environments and the natural world, and partially regulated by certain elements in our daily routine. The wide variation that we see in human circadian rhythms is interesting—we're not totally sure exactly why people have different genetic variations when it comes to circadian rhythm, but we can certainly take some guesses as to why we might have evolved to have different preferences of awakeness, perhaps having to do with geography, climate, or vigilance and security. Plus, there may be other reasons, not related to sleep, that circadian rhythms vary: circadian clocks play a role in many other processes, including metabolism, which I mentioned above, but also the *immune system*. One thing sleep and circadian scientists are particularly interested in figuring out right now is how to harness circadian rhythms to positively impact the immune system. For example: because metabolism is hooked to the circadian clock, we suspect that some people may have better responses to medications when taken at certain circadian phases rather than others. There is now an entire field of study surrounding this: *chronomedicine*. If we can better understand each individual's circadian rhythm, including in their cells and organs, more precisely, we may be able to treat people in a more personalized way.[3]

Your circadian rhythm is a foundational biological process that unfolds inside you at the chemical and cellular level, and which impacts so much about your sleep, your health, and your overall experience of life. So how much of it *is* actually within your control, and how much do you just have to live with?

## Can We "Reset" Our Circadian Rhythms?

A man—let's call him Ben—called the clinic out of the blue one day. He'd come across a fun video I'd done a short time before for *Wired* magazine—they had a whole series where experts in various fields explained their work to people at various levels of comprehension. My video started with me explaining sleep to a very smart eight-year-old kid, and ended with me struggling to keep up with a highly trained neuroscientist! Ben found the video when he was searching a little desperately for a solution to his sleep problem. He told me he had an unusual natural sleep cycle where he'd be awake all night, and asleep all day, like a nocturnal animal. It had been this way for years. He'd tried to move his sleep and wake times, but his body just seemed to boomerang back to this pattern. Over time, he'd figured out ways to manage it. But his main tactic was pretty extreme: Every few weeks, he would stay up for forty-eight hours straight to "reset" himself so he could be awake during the day for important events related to his work. He wanted to know: could I help him?

Ben had what we call a "phase delay," and a pretty severe one at that. A phase delay is, essentially, when your circadian rhythm is not in line with the rest of the world. Some people are night owls by nature (*delayed sleep phase* is the technical term), but this guy was maybe the most extreme night owl I'd ever encountered. He was forty-five years old, and according to him, had had this condition for his whole life.

I asked him if his work was compatible with his phase delay—nope. He worked for a big insurance company that required a nine-to-five schedule; he constantly found himself watching the clock, wondering how he was going to get through the day. His "reset" every few weeks would help briefly, but staying up for two straight days was a huge strain. And I was worried about the long-term effects—we now know that short sleepers are more at risk for all kinds of poor health outcomes, including heart disease, obesity, depression, and even Alzheimer's and dementia.[4]

Here's what I told Ben: "There's a few things we can do. We can try light therapy in the mornings. Melatonin supplements at night. There's a stimulant called *modafinil*, which is often used to treat shift-work disorder and patients with hypersomnia, that we can use to help you stay alert when your brain and body want to be sleeping. We could do chronotherapy—that's when we push you the other direction and sleep deprive you until you *want* to go to sleep at the right time—basically what you are already doing with your 'reset' strategy. If we're diligent about it, we may be able to slowly shift your schedule. But to be honest with you, it may not work very well in your situation. It might be the case that this world was not made for you."

Sounds harsh, I know. It never feels good delivering this kind of news to someone who is suffering. But at the same time, I like to emphasize that it's not the patient's fault. It's the world that's being inflexible.

I wanted to give Ben options: if he wanted to try the hard path forward to correct his phase delay, I was willing to try. But people who have this severe of a phase delay often cope in different ways, like opting into jobs they can do at night. I've treated people with significant phase delays and circadian rhythm disorders, and in a lot of cases they've worked nocturnal jobs, or very flexible jobs. I see a disproportionate number of people who've opted into overnight jobs like security guards or computer programmers. Sometimes it works really well for them, but a fair number of people who experience severe phase delays experience depression—they don't have the same experiences other people do, and it can be lonely.

"We can try some of these interventions," I told Ben, "but going into it I want you to know that you might be fighting this forever. In the long term, you may want to consider a different job."

In the end, Ben took a mixed approach—he worked on shifting his circadian rhythm enough so that he could live some of his life during the daylight hours, but he also took a disability leave and started considering his options for a career that might be more in line with his genetic predisposition to being at his best, most alert, wakeful self at night.

However, please know that this extreme of a phase delay is extremely uncommon—in fact, the reported prevalence of delayed sleep phase syndrome is less than 0.2 percent of the general population.[5] (In adolescents, that spikes up to as high as 15 percent—but it's transient, meaning not permanent.[6]) What's much more typical is that people who find themselves in this sort of pattern—up at night, sleepy during the day—have behavioral factors that are reinforcing it. Folks I see in the clinic (and, I'll admit it, myself) often engage in things later that keep them up: social media, gaming, work, reading, and hobbies that they feel they don't have time for during the day. I see this a lot with artists: they get deeply involved in a project and suddenly, it's 3 a.m.

Most of us don't have a phase delay like Ben. We have behaviors that we engage in, for lots of valid reasons, that perpetuate a sleep struggle. We have interests we can't get to during the day, we have work pressures, we have kids with their own sleep struggles. But then, a lack of structure around our *wake* time compounds the problem, keeping our dysregulated sleep cycle rolling along. We're up late working, hooked into a project, caring for a baby, and we end up sleeping in when we can to "catch up." Then that day, we can't build up enough sleep pressure to fall asleep earlier, and the cycle continues.

This is where zeitgebers come in. To a point, your circadian rhythm is genetic, yes. But it's malleable. It *will* respond to pressures from the environment and your routine. Factors like when you wake, when drink your coffee or tea, when you eat and exercise, and what you do routinely before bed as a "trigger" for bedtime, can press on your circadian rhythm and shift it. Just think about the last time you traveled somewhere—whether it was a two-hour time change or a twelve-hour one—and how you coped. I'm guessing that you immediately tried to align your schedule with the clock in the new location. (If you didn't, then try this next time!) Without thinking about it, you started eating breakfast in the morning when you usually do; dinner when you usually do; maybe even a walk or an exercise class when you usually do. Maybe you dragged yourself out of bed the second day, even though you still wanted to sleep because your body was hours behind. If you did all those things, you may have found that you bounced back from jet lag rather quickly. Within a couple days, your wake and sleep times (your internal clock) were well matched to your new, external clock. That's an example of you adjusting your circadian rhythm. You put pressures on it using these "levers" within your routine; it responded.

When people come into my clinic, the *first thing* I tell them to do is to pick a wake-up time and stick to it—seven days a week. I start with this first because it's the number-one most effective thing that most people can do to solve their sleep struggles. Consistency is key—your body craves it, and it can have powerful effects. And yet, a lot of folks struggle with it. It can be a hard adjustment to make. We're always trying to "game the system" for that day, that night. You have a bad night of sleep? You'll sleep in longer to make up the loss. It seems logical. But it's actually the worst thing you can do.

## Stop Giving Yourself Jet Lag on Purpose!

If you get up at 6 a.m. some days, and then other days at 9, you're throwing off your circadian rhythm. You're putting yourself, intentionally, into a state of jet lag. It's as if you're flying through three time zones every Saturday, trying to acclimate, and then flying back.

A lot of patients I work with come in and say, "I *know* I'm supposed to get up at the same time every day, but . . ." *I just can't. It's too hard. I'm too tired. My work schedule is unpredictable.* I get it. And honestly, if you're not in a struggle with sleep, maybe sleeping in on the weekend is perfectly fine. Just like that extra glass of wine, slice of pizza, or scoop of ice cream, it can be a delicious indulgence that makes life worth living. But if you're in my clinic (or maybe, reading this book) it means things aren't going so well on the sleep front. If that's the case, then this stable wake time is really something you need to try. So when patients have a million reasons why it won't work, here's what I say to them:

**The time you choose is up to you**. When people come into the lab, I say, "If you had to commit to a time, what would it be?" Answer that question right now. I'm not going to dictate that you have to wake up early, or any particular time at all. Find a time that works with your schedule—if you can manage work, kids, whatever else you have going on, then it's a great time to wake up as far as I'm concerned. Once you've decided, set an alarm. Alarms can come in lots of forms. I have young kids, so I have human alarms. (They're pretty expensive though, so I wouldn't suggest them if you're only trying to solve this problem.)

**Don't stress—there's wiggle room.** If you set your time at 8 a.m., and wake up at 8:15 one Saturday, it's not going to ruin all your progress. A little flexibility and forgiveness is OK. This is about consistency in the big picture. Mostly what I want is for you to make the effort.

**Make it worth it.** Sometimes, sticking to this is a little painful. You may be moving your wake-up time earlier as you begin to stabilize your sleep cycles—especially on your days off, if you're used to sleeping in. Those are going to be the hardest days to stick to this commitment. So reward yourself, immediately, when you get up. This is a classic lesson from behavior change, and it works.

One guy I worked with wanted to improve his sleep, but was really struggling with the idea of the same wake-up time every day. He wanted to sleep in. It felt good to sleep in. He believed his body needed the recovery time. But it was keeping his circadian rhythm confused and his sleep drivers dysregulated. So, we workshopped a new plan. He'd get up with the alarm, and then immediately walk to the coffee shop near his home and order his favorite drink: a dry cappuccino. It ended up being this lovely quiet time for him, away from the house with its myriad responsibilities, away from the demands of kids and family. He'd read the paper, which he never usually found time to do. The extra time he'd carved out, because he kept his wake-up time consistent, felt like a gift.

Another woman I worked with decided to walk down to the beach near her house—it became a morning ritual, and something she found she looked forward to as soon as her eyes opened to the beeping alarm—she was happy to get up. Other people have used different tactics: Preparing a hot breakfast when they usually just quickly eat cereal. Making coffee and playing a sudoku puzzle. Taking a long, energizing shower. Just going out on the porch to enjoy the sunrise.

**And finally, picture that sleep balloon.** Remember the balloon analogy here. The minute you wake up, that "sleep pressure" begins, slowly, to build. If you get the sleep you need, it's flat when you wake up—no matter what time you wake up, whether it's 6 a.m. or noon. Starting from that moment, the balloon gradually inflates. For an easier, more effortless, more natural sleep experience, start inflating that balloon at roughly the same time every day.

## Less Chaos, More Calm

This new level of structure in the mornings can be really helpful for people. When we have a little more predictability, other things begin to get more predictable, too. When life feels chaotic, providing clear markers of when certain activities (like sleep) start and stop can let your brain subconsciously track and compartmentalize stuff a little better. By keeping a stable wake time, you remove some of the uncertainty and randomness from the morning. And as you stick to it, you may find that your days feel looser and less frantic. You begin to be able to find more time within your busy schedule for things you enjoy—a beneficial ripple effect of stabilizing your sleep drivers.

Life can feel like jet lag if our two sleep drivers are out of alignment. And you don't want to spend months or weeks of your life living in jet lag—with cognitive fog, a less-efficient metabolism, difficulties coping with stress, and more. But this also shows us *exactly* how to treat this problem, and reminds us how adaptable we are. How long does it typically take you to adjust from jet lag—a day or two? A week? You can do this in the same amount of time.

TODAY'S PRACTICE

# PICK YOUR TIME AND STICK TO IT

We don't *make* sleep happen; sleep comes to us. So, we can't choose a time to fall asleep, and it's essential that we don't put that kind of pressure on ourselves at night when trying to improve our sleep. But we can powerfully influence when we fall asleep through when we wake up. And when we wake is absolutely within our control. So starting today, we're going to begin stabilizing and regulating our circadian rhythm and homeostatic sleep drive.

*Your Mission for Today*

1. *Pick your time!* Choose a wake-up time you can consistently maintain every day of the week, including the weekend (or whenever your days off may be). You'll want to choose a time that suits your life, and if possible, your preprogrammed preference. Because each of us has a certain sleep need each night (usually at least seven hours for an adult), once this wake-up time is established, you'll soon begin to notice yourself feeling sleepy around the same time each night.

2. *Set your alarm!* Program your alarm or phone for your chosen time now—for every day this week. Some people don't want to use an alarm; they prefer to wake up naturally. That's great, if you're in the habit of waking

up at a particular time and you don't need to adjust. But if your body's dysregulated, you're not going to be able to pull that off. Give yourself the digital assist. If you stick to your plan long enough, you may cease to need it.

3. ***Get some light!*** As soon as you wake up, get up and open the blinds. If it's feasible (and not too cold!), go right outside. If you're trying to shift your wake-up time, light exposure is a powerful zeitgeber that can jump-start your system.

4. ***Reward yourself for waking up.*** Make a nice cup of coffee. Read a book. Take a walk. Put on some music. Take a long hot shower. Pick something that you can look forward to, that you may not always be able to find time for in a typical hectic morning. Teach your brain and body that getting up every day is more rewarding than sleeping in. It will internalize this message.

5. ***And finally . . .*** Take a moment to fill out your sleep diary! It will take less than a minute of your time this morning, and we'll need the data later this week.

## Troubleshooting

### Strategies to Try If You're Encountering Challenges

- ***If you keep snoozing . . .*** Put the alarm clock across the room. Force yourself to get up in order to turn it off! The odds you get back in bed are much slimmer. Long term, consider investing in an alarm clock that gradually increases the light in the room. Many of my patients find it to be a gentle yet effective way to wake up.

- **Make sure your reward is really rewarding!** Some people try to "reward" themselves with something like an exercise class—believing they *should* enjoy it or that it will be beneficial in the long term. And they're right—it would be beneficial in the long term! But they also end up sleeping in if exercise is actually something they're dreading. Maybe save the exercise for later. Choose something that's really a reward for you. Don't try to optimize or take advantage of this time: your assignment is to give yourself a real treat this morning, and every morning that you hit your goal.

# DAY 2

# EASE OFF THE GAS

**HOW MANY TIMES HAVE YOU FELT STRESSED SO FAR TODAY?**

If your answer is *zero*, you're lucky—and rare! You might be a Zen master. More likely, you fall into the same category as most of us on planet Earth, with days full of ups and downs that start pretty much as soon as you open your eyes, and your brain starts whirring. I know that on busy days, as soon as I'm out of bed, I'm already ticking through everything I've got coming up: getting the kids to school, all the tasks I have to do before I get to the lab, all the tasks I have to do once I *do* get to the lab.

A busy day can feel like a minefield, with countless small triggers that can raise your blood pressure and set off an explosion of stress. So how much will this affect you tonight, when you finally slide between the sheets, close your eyes, and wait for sleep to sweep you away? Will the stress of the day get in your way?

## Understanding the Sleep-Stress Link

Sleep and stress are deeply intertwined. And this intersection between *sleep* and *stress* is actually where I do the work I'm most passionate about. Your body's stress response, and how you manage stress, can impact your sleep. But even more powerfully, your sleep determines how well you handle stress. It's a cyclical relationship. So let's take a dive into the relationship between sleep and stress, so you can understand how to step out of a cycle that may be sabotaging your sleep.

You know your own body's stress response. Consider how many times a day you feel that spike as your system responds to a stressful stimulus. It may feel like your stress response is getting switched on over and over again throughout the day at the slightest trigger. You know the feeling: that flare of worry and anxiety, that intrusive thought that pops into your brain without warning, your body tensing up as stress hormones swirl into your bloodstream. Is every hit of that stress cocktail knocking another hour off your sleep tonight? Maybe, but you might be surprised to learn that even if your days are stress-heavy, stress itself may not always be the problem.

Our systems are remarkably good at processing stress, and the stressful experiences we have during the day may stay with us at bedtime less than you might imagine. Studies we've run in our sleep lab (along with many other studies run elsewhere) have discovered that our daytime experience of stress is *not* always a great predictor of sleep.[1] In fact, you can have a really high-stress day followed by a great night of sleep. There are a couple of exceptions: First, if the stressful event happens close to bedtime (like if you get into an argument with your partner or get some bad news right as you're winding down) that will certainly impact your ability to shut your brain off for the night. And second, if the stressor is severe (if you get fired or get in a car accident first thing in the morning), well, that'll probably affect you that night! But that's not reflective of a typical day. Overall, your mind and body can cope quite well with everyday stress—even when it feels intense. For instance, *peak and recovery* stress (where your body mounts a stress response, but then comes back to physiological baseline after) is something your system was built for, and can even be healthy for your cells—it triggers a cleanup process where the body sheds old, damaged, or senescent (dead) cells.

The point here isn't that stress is never going to be a problem for sleep—certain types of stress can become an issue, and we'll be talking about that shortly. What I want you to understand right from the beginning is that when it comes to the typical stress of your life—the ups and downs of your job, of parenting, of navigating the logistics of finances, family, and more—you are actually fairly resilient. One of the big things I see getting in people's way at night is *worry* that they won't be able to get a good night's sleep, or a belief that they are already doomed to a bad night's sleep. So even before we dive into what you can do about stress to set yourself up for success, I want to dispel any notion you might have that *stress = insomnia*. Don't get caught in the loop of thinking, "I was so stressed today, I'll never be able to fall asleep." Not true! So take comfort and confidence in this area of the science: today's stress will not preclude you from getting great sleep.

Data from research studies that capture participants' daily stress and nightly sleep for days on end actually indicate that the stress-sleep impact runs more strongly in the *other* direction: poor sleep or short sleep makes you more vulnerable to stress.[2]

We did a study on stress and sleep in mothers who were caring for young children—as you may have intimately experienced, taking care of little kids is a scenario that's rife with potential stressors. We had two study groups: one was a group of moms who classified themselves as experiencing a lot of stress typically, the other group reported low stress going into the study. So, we had a "high stress" and a "low stress" group. We wanted to investigate how sleep impacted the experience of stress and how stress during the day affected their nights, capturing the sleep-stress cycle.

Participants kept a detailed "stress journal" where they recorded when and why they felt stress during the day, and also what event triggered it. Simultaneously, we tracked their sleep using research-grade wearables. We weren't surprised to find that people who slept less than they usually did experienced more stress the following day. It lined up with other studies we've run in our own lab, as well as research from others that shows that when people don't get enough sleep, they experience their days as more stressful.[3]

It makes sense: when you short-shrift your sleep, the cognitive impact on you is tangible and immediate. It's harder to regulate your emotions, control impulses, even pay attention and hold information in working memory. All of this will make your day more stressful than it would be otherwise. We've all had the experience of feeling fractured, unfocused, and reactive after a bad night of sleep. It's not the end of the world—bad nights of sleep happen! But if you're habitually sleep-deprived—even just a little—it's going to have an impact on how you experience your life.

Here's what was really interesting about that study with the sleep-deprived moms. We had participants write down *exactly* what it was that was stressful to them. Then, we took those diaries and handed them off to expert coders, who grouped these "stress triggers" into categories, determining as best they could how bad they were, really, in terms of how stressful they were. Were they significant stressors? Or minor hassles? Then they cross-referenced people's reactions with their sleep logs. What they found: *everybody* felt more stressed with empirically stressful events whether they had good sleep or poor sleep. If something stressful happened, then they felt, well, stressed. What bad sleep seemed to do was increase people's stress response to *low and moderate* stressors—or even to events that might not normally stress them out at all. Bad sleep lowered their threshold for what felt stressful.

## Short on Sleep, High on Stress

Skimping on sleep changes the way you perceive things. It changes your experience of life. Exactly how much it does is still a developing field of study, and something I've spent a ton of time researching in the lab, but one thing we do know is that under sleep deprivation, people experience events as more stressful than they would have if they'd had sufficient sleep. Their lens on the world is different.

Under periods of less sleep, we are more likely to get into conflicts, including with those we love the most—in one study, Dr. Amie Gordon, who is at the University of Michigan, found that when participants sleep worse than they typically do they reported more conflicts with their partner the following day.[4] Not necessarily surprising, but it gets even more interesting: in a second study, the researchers brought couples to the laboratory to participate in a task that focused on a conflict in their relationship—a hot topic, things like who does the dishes and the grocery shopping, balancing time for each other, politics, etc. The couple worked to resolve it, then completed questionnaires asking how they felt, how they thought their partner felt, and whether they thought they had successfully resolved the conflict. What they discovered: First, partners who slept poorly the night before felt more negative emotions and fewer positive emotions during the conflict. Second, the worse a partner slept, the worse they were in judging the emotions of their partner during the conflict—they showed less empathetic accuracy, an inability to put themselves in their partner's place. And finally, and perhaps the most concerning when it comes to sustaining a cordial relationship, having one partner report poor sleep significantly lowered the odds of conflict resolution. The takeaway? Your sleep has a huge impact on your relationships with the people closest to you.

Sleep loss can also do a number on our health behaviors, including dietary choices, leading us to make ones that may not be great for our sleep (or health) later on. In one of my favorite studies on sleep, stress, and the kinds of choices people make, researchers built a faux grocery store, fully stocked, and sent people off to shop in it. They gave them money to spend and free reign to choose what they wanted. Then they deprived people of sleep. The sleep-deprived shoppers chose different foods than they did when they were well rested: they filled their carts with more calorically dense products. Why? Something different was happening in the brain when they were short on sleep—researchers theorized that sleep deprivation may have increased what they call "hedonic drive," or even fueled feelings of hunger. In other lab-based studies, my colleague Dr. Matt Walker, who is across the Bay at UC Berkeley, deprived participants of sleep, then put them into an fMRI machine. An fMRI can track the flow of oxygenated blood as it moves through the brain; by doing so, it can see which areas of the brain have the most activity in response to certain stimuli. So with the magnet of the fMRI whirring, tracking brain activity, researchers showed people images of different foods and watched to see what would happen. What they saw was that the reward centers of their sleep-deprived brains were more "lit up" in response to high-sugar, high-fat foods compared to when they were well rested.[5]

What we think is happening is that with sleep deprivation, our capacity to *resist* those kinds of impulses and cravings that come from those lit-up areas in the brain drops. It's not just that our reward centers are "on overdrive," but also that our capacity to slow down and put the brakes on has diminished—the "brakes" in this scenario being your executive control system, or that "angel on your shoulder" that guides you to make the better, smarter, more strategic choices in any situation. Executive control makes sure your *goals* and *actions* are in alignment. And what we see with sleep deprivation in lab studies is that for these participants, that executive control basically "turns off." Short on sleep, we're all gas, no brakes.

This missing brake pedal is also why we think that sleep-deprived people are more sensitive to stress and have a harder time regulating their emotions, which translates into real-world consequences. We've seen, for example, that police officers with sleep disorders are more likely to experience uncontrolled anger toward a suspect.[6] Sleepy judges dole out longer prison sentences.[7] And in organizations with hierarchies, sleep-deprived supervisors are much more likely to behave poorly toward their subordinates.[8] In general, we see that sleep-deprived people get turned inward, laser-focused on their own needs, as opposed to the needs of the larger group or community. In short: when we aren't getting enough sleep, we are not our best selves.

To make matters worse, when we experience our lives as stressful and difficult (as we do when we're short on sleep) we make certain decisions to cope with that stress that sabotage us later on. We have a late coffee. Another drink. We soothe our stress by consuming certain foods and substances. Under stress, we make the same kinds of food choices that we do under sleep loss: we crave fatty and sugary foods. And it's no accident.

There's a biological reason that our bodies are crying out for this kind of stuff when our stress response is churning: *because it dampens the cortisol response*. When you have a high cortisol response going on, your body prefers these high-fat, high-sugar substances because they act as a kind of "medicine" for stress.[9] But they're not great for our bodies, and often, not great for our sleep.

Sleep researchers had been aware for some time that there was a link between shorter sleep and consuming higher amounts of certain foods, like processed carbs and sugar; meanwhile people who ate more plants and fiber seemed to sleep better. But was this correlation or causation? The researcher Dr. Marie-Pierre St-Onge, who is at Columbia University, has worked toward untangling this web. Along with her colleagues, she ran a study[10] where she strictly controlled the sleep and diet conditions: researchers monitored people's sleep (as opposed to having them self-report) and a nutritionist prepared their meals. The results echoed previous findings: a diet heavier on plants and healthy fats was indeed associated with better sleep. But here, they discovered the reason: when people drifted away from their high-fiber, fruit-and-veggie-heavy diet and toward saturated fats and simple carbohydrates, they experienced a *reduction in slow-wave sleep*. Slow-wave sleep is believed to be the phase of your sleep cycle where you get your deep, restorative sleep.

Carb lovers, pay attention here: carbs are an interesting case. Studies have unearthed that while most carbohydrates will actually help you fall asleep faster, only certain types will help you *stay* asleep. Simple and sugary carbs (think pizza, white bread, bagels, pasta) can cause more wake ups throughout the night. In contrast, complex carbs (again, these are the more high-fiber foods like sweet potatoes, oatmeal, and whole grains) can stabilize your sleep patterns—possibly, Dr. St-Onge theorizes, because they also stabilize your blood sugar.[11]

The moral here: the foods your brain and body cry out for when you're stressed, and which you're most likely to reach for during those times, may indeed be making it harder for you to stay asleep and to get good sleep.

To wrap up: People who have been sleep deprived—even just a little—perceive the world as more stressful. They make choices under stress that they might not have otherwise, and that may not be conducive to their next night of sleep—stuff like food selections, skipping exercise because of time pressure, and more. They experience a biological stress response to events that they otherwise wouldn't. They may even "select into" more stressful experiences. And there's a biological cost to this. Stress, we now know, when it's constant, ages you at the cellular level. It wears down your telomeres, the protective caps at the ends of your chromosomes that play a significant role in determining the cellular aging of your body.[12] And guess what? Insufficient sleep does that, too.[13]

If you experience insomnia or have been struggling to get enough sleep, this may be frustrating to hear. *I know sleep is important,* you might be yelling, *that's why I'm reading this book!* But there are a couple important reasons why I'm going into it here.

### It Offers Us a Way to Intervene

As I said before, sleep and stress are cyclical. Short, more-disrupted sleep leads to higher stress; the choices we make under high stress can lead to poorer sleep. Each perpetuates the other. But when we see exactly how the arrows point in both directions, and *which* choices we make under stress most affect us, we can step into this cycle and begin to neutralize it.

It's actually good news: we have two opportunities for intervention. If we can improve sleep a little, we can bring down our overall level of stress. And if we can regulate the stress response, or at the very least become aware of some of the things we're doing in *response* to stress, we may see some sleep benefits. You get spillover in both directions.

When I work with people in our sleep clinic, I find a lot of success with this approach: wiggle the needle a little bit in each direction. And just as the sleep-stress cycle can be exponentially damaging, it can be exponentially *beneficial* when you use it to your advantage. The less stressed you are, the more you can stick to daytime choices that don't undermine sleep. The more sleep you get, the more capacity you have to make those choices. Once you get it going, the momentum can be exponential, like a stone rolling down a hill, picking up speed.

### You Might Need to Change Your Life

A lot of people who come into my clinic with insomnia discover that there is something baked into their lifestyle that is incompatible with good sleep. This is a harder challenge to overcome, especially when you're locked into a particular job, for example, or when the pressures affecting you are completely out of your control: the economy, or maybe a loved one who is ill. I won't pretend that every obstacle is possible to remove. But it's worth considering that we live in a society where we've glamorized short sleep and long work hours, and this is a huge factor for a lot of people I see. We elevate productivity and devalue rest. Which is ironic, because *rest* is what we most need in order to be productive, creative, effective, innovative.

Across the board, people are getting insufficient sleep. Frankly, it's an epidemic. And our sleep challenges don't exist in a vacuum, outside of this context. What I see in the clinic is that we sometimes misdiagnose the cause. We believe we have a sleep problem, when, really, we have a life problem.

## A Life Problem?

Your sleep is your well of resilience. It's what provides you with the armor you need for the slings and arrows that life flings at you. So if there's something in your life that's causing enough stress that it's chronically disrupting your capacity to get the sleep you need, we need to deal with it. In the sleep clinic, I end up in conversations like these all the time. When people come in, they submit extensive questionnaires and keep detailed diaries of their days and their nights. And when we analyze them and begin working with these folks to improve their sleep, we frequently discover that there's no medical or biological basis for their short sleep. Instead, there are knots in their lifestyle somewhere that are initially hard to see, but that need to be untangled.

At the beginning of this chapter, I told you that your brain and body were built for handling normal daytime stress and meeting challenges, and that's true. We have all these things going for us: your homeostatic sleep drive and circadian rhythms are powerful. You have these innate tools working for you that you don't even have to worry about—personally, I take a lot of solace in knowing that, and trusting it. But under higher levels of stress, we're all susceptible to sleep disruptions, and those natural sleep processes do start to have trouble tipping the balance into dreamland. In these cases, we *do* need to intervene.

There are two major things that can be in play with higher levels of stress getting in the way of sleep: *cortisol* and *the sympathetic nervous system.*

The stress you experience affects the release of cortisol in your blood stream. Cortisol is a metabolic hormone: it ensures that there's adequate glucose for your cells to use. Essentially, cortisol helps regulate energy.

You have cortisol ebbing and flowing in your body at all times, and it has its own circadian rhythm, irrespective of stress—it's a normal, healthy part of your body's processes. The normal fluctuation of cortisol influences the availability of glucose when your brain or muscles need it. In other words, demand for energy triggers the release of cortisol. And *stress* is one of those triggers. Your body wants to make more energy available, and *fast* (think fight-or-flight response and how this would aid your survival: a tiger's staring you down and you need to run!) so it gives you a "shot" of cortisol. Now, as I said earlier, typical daily stressors (traffic, a negative interaction, a high-pressure work situation) will probably not affect your sleep. Your body will begin to gradually metabolize that cortisol after the stressful event passes and basically, that's it. The exception is if you're experiencing frequent stress triggers and consistently elevated cortisol. That starts to become a problem for sleep.

Cortisol is also part of your *awakening* response. There's a cortisol spike that happens right as you wake up—your body's way of giving you a little push into consciousness and out of bed to start the day. You have a peak of cortisol in the early morning, a little burst of energy to get you moving—for the most part, it decreases through the rest of the day. By the early evening, your body should be in a low-cortisol state, so that you'll be ready to drift off in the next couple hours. But for people under chronic stress, we see that their cortisol levels don't dip the same way. They stay high.

For a lot of people, even with elevated cortisol they'll be able to fall asleep—the homeostatic sleep drive and circadian rhythm are powerful pressures, and they can overcome a lot. But it is possible that elevated cortisol across the day and into the evening can impact your sleep onset and be associated with poorer sleep. We know that people who receive high doses of steroids (like prednisone) are frequently pushed into insomnia; cortisol is actually a natural steroid.

Constantly elevated cortisol is an example of what we might call "a dysregulated stress physiology." The other example of this is an overactive *sympathetic nervous system*. In a healthy, balanced system, there's an appropriate toggling that happens between the sympathetic nervous system (fight, flight, freeze) and the parasympathetic nervous system (rest and digest). In order to sleep, we need the parasympathetic to take over. But for people whose stress system is dysregulated, their hyper arousal system stays "on" in response, making it hard to let go and relax. Blood pressure is higher. Heart rate variability (HRV), which correlated with slow-wave sleep, is lower.

If we're carrying around a lot of stress, it's hard to disengage the sympathetic and amp up the parasympathetic at bedtime— we're just *on*, we feel wired not tired. And it doesn't have to be some catastrophic stressor for this to happen: just the simple stress of working right up until bedtime can cause this. The energy that's required (both in terms of cortisol production and the engagement of the sympathetic nervous system) is just not compatible with sleep.

So, back to my question: What in your life is standing in the way of good sleep? What's causing stress? And what can you do about it?

I had a patient who came into the clinic with a complaint of insomnia. She couldn't fall asleep at night and struggled to wake up in the morning in time for work. She worked in finance, cared deeply about doing well at her job, and was concerned about her lack of sleep impacting her performance. The first thing we did (which we always do) is rule out medical conditions that might be the root cause of the insomnia, but she didn't have any complicating factors. She was young and healthy. But when she completed the sleep diaries I sent her home with, it revealed that her sleep was really bad. She wasn't getting enough of it, for one thing. And it was extremely unstructured. She'd sleep right until her alarm (6:45 a.m.) most days, but worked long hours, stayed up late, and then struggled to fall asleep once she was in bed, worrying about how fast she needed to fall asleep in order to get enough rest. When she could, she'd go to bed really early to "make up" for the sleep that she'd lost. The same was true on the weekends, sleeping in until late morning.

The problem with this: her sleep was unpredictable. Her body didn't know *what* time to fall asleep; nor was she giving herself any real wind-down time at the end of the day. When your sleep schedule—and your *day* schedule—is unstructured, your body doesn't know what's coming. It doesn't get the cues it needs to turn down the stress system and turn up the melatonin. Confused about what it's supposed to be doing at any given time, your system doesn't wind down and prepare for sleep—it just keeps going with the shots of energy-producing cortisol, keeping you energized for the workday it believes is still happening.

"You don't have a nighttime problem," I told her. "You have a daytime problem."

*Insomnia* is an interesting thing. There's no blood test I can do to tell you if you have insomnia or not. We diagnose it largely through self-reporting: if people say they regularly aren't sleeping well (trouble falling or staying asleep at least three nights per week for the past three months) and feel terrible despite having the opportunity to sleep, and it can't be explained by substances or another medical or psychiatric condition, then there's your diagnosis. And so the cure is, similarly, both vague but often surprisingly easy to arrive at. When people start to feel better, start sleeping better, and stop worrying about their sleep, then they're in remission. Sometimes that means they're sleeping better, longer, or deeper. Other times it means their sleep has simply become more predictable and less effortful, with less anxiety surrounding it. And for many, many people who come into the clinic for help with insomnia, their real problem is a mismanaged day: their days are too packed with stress and activity. Their days are unpredictable because they're busy. They skip meals one day, stay up late another. Without those cues (*zeitgebers*, as we discussed on day one) their minds and bodies, at bedtime, are at sea. They're treating sleep as an afterthought, which is ironic because most patients with insomnia will tell me that they spend way too much time thinking about their sleep (or lack thereof).

With this particular patient, we began by coming up with a loose schedule that she'd stick to: there was wiggle room, but she really had to try to hit the same beats every day in terms of when she woke, ate, exercised, and shut down her computer at night. What this immediately revealed was that her work was so demanding, it was regularly eating into her ability to go to bed and protect the time for sleep. It was really hard for her to make this shift—she had deadlines to meet with real consequences if she missed them. It didn't feel like there was any give. But one critical thing to understand is that sleep debt makes you less effective. It dampens your capacity for quick and creative thinking. You have more struggles with attention and focus; you become slower and less efficient. It's counterintuitive but true: sometimes the best way to get something urgent done is to *not* do it right that second—if "right that second" is late at night and way past your bedtime.

I told this patient that she needed to reevaluate. "I can't help you with this part," I said. "Figure out a way to make more time for sleep—or accept that within this lifestyle, you're going to be short on sleep, and live with it the best you can."

The intervention in the end, for her, was that she had to get a different job. And she did! She ended up making a lateral move to a different company that was less rigid and more holistically focused on the wellness and vitality of its employees.

Don't worry—you probably don't need to get a different job! But if you try all the tactics in this book and are still really struggling, it's worth thinking about whether something in your life needs to change. A chronic sleep problem can be a canary in the coal mine that something is off—and that it's not (only) about your bedtime routine. If you are regularly shorting your sleep because of high-stress days and/or a rigid and demanding work life, it's worth a second look. Because as this patient discovered, sleep debt is cumulative—it builds up across the week as we shortchange night after night. And even though it seems we should be able to "make up" that sleep in the same way, by sleeping in extra when we have the chance, it unfortunately doesn't work that way. You can't make up sleep; you can't save up sleep.

I don't mean this to sound grim—if you have a rough night and don't get much sleep, your body will very likely compensate the next day. You'll wake up with your sleep balloon already slightly inflated; you may take a nap or go to bed early. All of that is perfectly OK, and nothing to stress about. What I'm talking about here is *chronic*, habitual sleep deprivation due to your routine, habits, or work demands. At social events I constantly hear people talking about how they'll "catch up on sleep this weekend," and I have to sit there silently knowing that's not how it works, and that they'll just end up confusing their circadian rhythm and entering the same cycle of late nights and tired days the following week.

However, before you go making any drastic moves, try some simple strategies first. These are tactics that anybody can wedge into their day—no matter how busy.

## Fixing Your Daytime Problem

In the NBA, athletes (and their coaches) know that they can only play a certain number of minutes per game if they're going to get through the season in fighting shape. They call this *load management*. We all need to think about load management in our own lives when it comes to how we pace our days.

The woman I mentioned earlier (who ended up switching

jobs for a more sustainable life) is typical of a lot of people I see in the clinic. They're busy and time-pressured, pushed to their limits by some combination of work, family obligations, or other responsibilities. They're carrying a lot of sleep debt. They may even be engaging (consciously or not) in something that we've started calling *revenge bedtime procrastination*, which is when people choose to stay up later than they should in an effort to take back some time for themselves after a day completely filled with obligations and to-do's. Revenge bedtime procrastination is a relatively new term, but it inspired a spate of articles and even scientific studies as people everywhere seemed to identify with the problem. Psychologists and researchers looking at the phenomenon believe that revenge bedtime procrastination happens when people need to exert control over their time— when their overly packed days are out of their control, chasing one to-do to the next, they take back their time at night.

Maybe your struggle after a busy day is that your stress is still high. Maybe it's that within a negative, exponential cycle of short sleep leading to a higher experience of stress, you're making choices during the day that sabotage sleep. Maybe it's that your day feels out of control, and so you're trying to reclaim some personal time late at night. Regardless, the fix is the same: *take breaks*. Real breaks. They can be short, but they should be screen-free, phone-free, and something that's relaxing, refreshing, or joyful. I'm not going to tell you exactly what to do: this varies by individual. But it's what I tell my patients who come into the sleep clinic. I say: This is your prescription. Make it happen, and *be militant about it*. Think of it like a medication I'm ordering you to take: no excuses.

Breaks can be short: five, ten, fifteen minutes—however long you've got. But take them. Take a lunch break. Take a walk. Get a coffee and drink it in the sun. Set a timer and meditate. Some people hate hearing advice to meditate—it does seem to be everywhere these days—but there's a reason for that. *It works*. Research shows that mindfulness meditation can provide some of the same restorative benefits as sleep does. How do we know? It turns out that people who meditate regularly (and who have done so long-term) also get less sleep at night.[14] The theory: they may actually need less sleep, due to processes in the brain during meditation that mimic certain processes during sleep. Meditation, for many, may relieve stress, and it may offer a small dose of the same kind of restoration you get with sleep.

In short: you cannot just *go go go* all day long. We can't go full tilt all day long and then switch off at night. The body doesn't work that way; the brain doesn't work that way. How you *live* during the day is where these issues originate—it's why we end up with high cortisol, an overactive sympathetic nervous system, or a subconscious desire to stay up too late. So give yourself a little restoration. A little goes a *long* way. And keep in mind that it might take a few days for you to see the impact: remember, we are wiggling the settings a little bit in each direction. Think of it like bringing down your "stress thermometer"—you don't let it get as high during the day, and then at bedtime, you don't have as far to go to drop the temperature back down. We drop that temperature a little and it gets a little easier to get good sleep; we get a little bit more sleep and it gets a little easier to manage our days and keep the temp low. It might not happen overnight, but just as the cyclical nature of the sleep-stress cycle can work against you, it can also work *for* you.

TODAY'S PRACTICE

# STRESS-BUSTING MICRO BREAKS

Today, take the long view about the day . . . and the week ahead. Look at the week as a whole. Think about how you might space out your responsibilities so that everything's not loaded into one time frame. And remember that one of your responsibilities is to yourself: *to make time for sleep, and for breaks*. This can help you plan and set doable expectations around deadlines and other big to-do's for yourself and others.

You can only accomplish so much. Pace yourself today, and all week long, with the idea of protecting your sleep time, and keeping that "stress thermometer" at a manageable level. If you don't get too wound up today, it'll be a lot easier to wind down later tonight.

Remember that in any given day, there will be unending demands for your time. Look ahead at the day the best you can and start now to reduce your likelihood of sleep debt. There's no banking sleep; you can't save it up. You can have some success making it up, but the deeper you get into sleep debt, the more difficult that becomes.

Today, we start making an important mental shift toward prioritizing sleep. We have this idea that "sleep doesn't put money in the bank." But *it does*. It sets you up to be successful. It's just one of the more invisible forces that does this—it's hard to see it. We acclimate to being tired, to operating at a deficit. We simply don't realize how much more effective and engaged we can be when we give ourselves a real shot at getting this essential restorative medicine every night.

And that means padding the day with downtime.

Chronically activated stress is hard to turn off at nighttime. We put too much pressure on nighttime strategies to undo the perils of the day. You need to take time *during* the day, to find moments of relaxation, restoration, and joy. Even the busiest days have their opportunities. Take them today.

## The Rules

Your goal today: Take 5 "micro breaks" during the day. They can be five, ten, or fifteen minutes long . . . or longer, if you have the bandwidth in your schedule.

To prepare: make a quick list of what you'll do on your breaks. Suggestions from me: A five-minute meditation (download an app like Headspace if you want some guidance). A ten-minute walk. Listening to fifteen minutes of your favorite podcast. Put on a favorite playlist and walk around the block; go outside and pull weeds in your garden in the sunshine, if that's something you find relaxing and satisfying. You choose: this is for you.

Choose one of these two ways of holding yourself accountable to your breaks:

1. *Set a timer.* Program five alarms into your phone to go off at times of your choosing. When the alarm goes off—to the extent that you can—drop what you're doing and do one of your break activities.

2. *"Anchor" your break to an existing staple in your routine.* Behavior scientists suggest this tactic as a quick and effective way to add a new element to your routine. Tether your break to something you do routinely. So, you might say, every time I go to the bathroom, I'm going to take a break right after. Or every time I answer an email (this depends on how many emails you get!).

Commit to doing this every day this week! Do this today—but do it tomorrow, and the next day, too. Hopefully, by the end of this week, it'll be baked into your routine to the point where you're benefiting from it, and not suffering a time crunch. And as always, remind yourself that it's worth it: your sleep is an investment in your future productivity, creativity, and happiness.

# DAY 3

# ENERGIZE—BUT DO IT RIGHT

**HOW DO YOU USUALLY FEEL BY MIDAFTERNOON? DO YOU FEEL A BIT** tired? Do you yawn, glance at the clock, try to regain your focus? Maybe you're right in the thick of your workday—you still have a lot left to do. But your energy is super low. You wonder if it was the timing of your lunch; maybe it's because you didn't sleep well last night. Maybe you need a snack to boost your blood sugar. You consider another cup of coffee.

This valley of low energy we usually experience during midafternoon is perfectly natural. It's another preprogrammed part of your circadian rhythm. We talked about this extensively in the last chapter, so you know that your internal clock releases cortisol in the morning to jump-start you, and then hits you with a nightcap of melatonin in the evening to wind you down. But that internal clock of yours is ticking away for *all* of the twenty-four hours in your day and night. It's always up to something.

While everyone is of course a little different, most people

follow this basic pattern: after you wake, your alertness level begins to rise, reaching its peak a couple hours later. In the early afternoon (for most people, somewhere around 1 p.m.) your circadian rhythm begins to dip. Alertness and energy levels decline, reaching a low point somewhere around 3 p.m. Finally, they swoop back up and rise again, reaching a secondary peak in the early evening—the average time is around 6 p.m.—before declining once more.

Now, you know your own rhythms and can adjust these average times to more accurately reflect your own circadian rhythm. If you're a morning person, you're going to skew earlier; if you're a night owl, you'll skew later. But know this: that internal clock of yours is programmed to have these dips. So, to a certain degree, that afternoon lull and slowdown you feel is simply a baked-in human tendency, and just part of the biological cycle of your day.

However, if you are having sleep issues at night, this may also be when the ramifications of short sleep or poor sleep are catching up to you. Remember that sleep-pressure balloon that starts to inflate as soon as your eyes fly open? Well, if you're someone who has interrupted sleep, or who wakes up too early, that balloon might be pretty full by midafternoon. When we're getting overwhelmed with sleepiness in the middle of the day, or sluggish and low-energy to the point that it's affecting our capacity to enjoy the day or get done what we need to get done, we look to various strategies to boost us through the slump and make it through the day. Some of those strategies are great; others can potentially tank your sleep long before the sun even begins to set. So let's talk about the do's and don'ts of navigating that afternoon slump.

## The Life-Changing Magic of . . . Caffeine

Confession: I love coffee. I start every morning with a cup. When I sit down to focus on something important, I make another. When I'm feeling that energy dip and need a pick-me-up— coffee. I love an artisanal pour-over as much as the next San Franciscan, but I'm happy with a Keurig pod. I just want it to be hot, and for that sweet caffeine to hit my bloodstream and make its way up to my brain as fast as humanly possible. Meanwhile, I'm a sleep scientist. I've studied, up close and personally, the impact of caffeine on the brain, and on nighttime sleep cycles. I know *exactly* how it will interact chemically in my brain later on to interfere with my sleep processes. And still, I pour myself another cup.

Whether or not you're a coffee drinker like me, the world is awash in caffeine. It's in the tea and soda we drink. It's laced into snacks and candy. Surveys have found that roughly 85 percent of the U.S. population drinks at least one caffeinated beverage per day.[1] On the aggregate, we are caffeinated. We are *awake*. Maybe too awake.

It's nothing new. Humans have used caffeine as a stimulant basically as far back as recorded history exists. There are origin stories of the discovery of caffeine from all over the world. From China: legend has it that around 2740 BCE, the emperor, who liked to boil his drinking water to sterilize it, didn't notice when the wind blew leaves from a wild tea bush into his drink. He drank it and felt refreshed, so goes the myth. From Ethiopia: a goatherd noted that whenever his flock ate from a particular berry bush, they refused to go to sleep and seemed wired with energy; he reported his observations to the monks at the local monastery, who made a brew from the berries and found that it kept them awake through long nights of prayer. In what is now Mexico, the ancient Olmecs made a bitter energizing drink out of cacao beans, which would much later be turned into *chocolate* by colonizing invaders, who mixed it with sugar to make it more palatable. Thousands of years later, in the early 1800s, a German chemist named Folger von Starbuck (just kidding—his name was Friedlieb Ferdinand Runge) isolated the chemical behind the zing of energy that people got from consuming plants like tea, coffee beans, the kola nut, mate, and more . . . an alkaloid he named *caffeine* after the German word for coffee.

Today, coffee is one of the most-consumed beverages on the planet. The International Coffee Organization reported that the world consumed 166,346 sixty-kilogram bags of coffee between 2020 to 2021, which works out to be about *1.4 trillion cups*[2]—another arrow pointing to our culture of always on, always awake, always going. Right now, this very second that you read these words, people around the world are sipping down twenty-six thousand cups of coffee. Another second ticks by, another twenty-six thousand. Another second . . . You get the point.

Caffeine is the single most widely consumed psychoactive substance on earth—and it's 100 percent naturally occurring.

Researchers now believe that the various plants that evolved to produce caffeine, a type of alkaloid, did so for survival purposes: caffeinated leaves falling from the plant into the soil around it made the area less hospitable to competing plants; caffeine repels certain insects that might prey on the plants; and finally, there is a symbiotic relationship between animals and caffeinated plants. Bees that pollinate a caffeine-producing plant feel that lovely buzz and remember it, come back, and help it reproduce again; humans who fell into the thrall of caffeine cultivated and tended those plants. Really, humans and caffeine-producing plants have helped each other thrive. (I know it helps me thrive.)

And it's true—there's nothing bad for you about caffeine! In fact, it may actually be healthy. Studies have found that coffee contains various antioxidants and anti-inflammatory properties that may protect against disease; coffee drinking is also associated with a lower risk of illnesses like heart disease, Alzheimer's, and type 2 diabetes.[3] So if you, too, are a coffee enthusiast, or love to get your energizing burst of caffeine through green tea or an ice-cold Diet Coke, then here's some good news: I'm not going to tell you to stop. What I am going to tell you is to have a cutoff time. Because here's the deal: you can do everything else in this book perfectly, but if you still have caffeine in your system while you're trying to fall asleep, none of it's going to work.

When you take a sip of your favorite caffeinated beverage, here's what happens. Remember that substance in your brain called *adenosine*, the neurochemical that causes sleepiness?

Well, caffeine actually has a very similar chemical structure to adenosine. It's able to essentially "fool" your brain's adenosine receptors, blocking the uptake of adenosine. So adenosine will continue to build up . . . but the caffeine you consumed has bound itself to those adenosine receptors and cancelled any feelings of sleepiness. This makes it a great way to maintain some alertness when you need it. And people have relaxing rituals around coffee, tea, mate, and other beverages that are beneficial in other ways. But it doesn't stop that adenosine from building up—which means that when the caffeine does start to fade, you're going to have a "coffee crash."

That's when a lot of us reach for another cup. But check the clock: what time is it? Compared to other chemicals, caffeine has a fairly long half-life. *Half-life* is a term stolen from nuclear physics, where it's used to describe how long it takes for something radioactive to decay to half its original strength. In the case of caffeine, the question is: how long does it take for *half* of what you consumed to still be in your system? The half-life of caffeine is around six hours. So let's do the math. At 3 p.m., you get a grande Starbucks coffee, which has 330 mg of caffeine, to fight that afternoon dip. That means that at 9 p.m., you'll still have 165 mg of caffeine coursing through your system. That's roughly two shots of espresso. Even if you do manage to fall asleep with that much caffeine competing for adenosine in your brain, you may end up having more restless, less restorative sleep: the chemistry of your sleep will be off.

The fix here is simple—be mindful of when you have your last caffeinated beverage. It can take up to ten hours for caffeine to completely clear your system. So count back from your bedtime and realize: caffeine is probably not the best strategy for boosting yourself through the late afternoon circadian dip. I try to be good about this myself, and I have been known to look at the clock and pour out my coffee. Tragic, but necessary.

## So What About a Nap?

Some people I've worked with during the COVID-19 pandemic have reported one silver lining: the ability to nap after they have a bad night of sleep. When you're working from home, it's a lot easier to hit the couch, close your eyes, and drop off to dreamland in the afternoon when you feel that wave of sleepiness. And because of the more flexible hours many now have (a double-edged sword, of course, as people have seen their start and end times for work creep earlier into the morning and later at night), it's more possible. But is it a good idea?

Data are emerging that during the pandemic, for some people, sleep *quantity* actually went up—perhaps because the erasure of commutes made sleeping in a little bit easier. However, at the same time, sleep *quality* went down.[4] People were getting more sleep, yes, but it was interrupted, restless, and less restorative, perhaps due to the spike in stress, anxiety, and depression that went hand-in-hand with the pandemic era, a time of intense uncertainty unlike anything most of us have ever been through. Ironically, people were suddenly able to actually get the recommended seven to nine hours—but putting in the hours wasn't enough. Sleep had to be restorative. For the "dishwasher of the brain" to really clear out all that metabolic waste and leave us feeling alert and refreshed, it has to go through all its cycles—just like a real dishwasher. Skipping or interrupting cycles, which happens more under stress, makes the whole process less effective. Strategies for dealing with interrupted sleep are coming up—for now, though, we need to get over this afternoon slump that can be exacerbated by poor quality sleep. So can you nap?

Sure! But do it right. Here's the deal with naps. They've been shown to boost alertness. The urge to nap can be a signal to your body that you really need to relieve some of that sleep pressure, and that you need a little more restoration in order to be at your cognitive peak and get through your day well. A nap can be really beneficial. The question is: Is it affecting your sleep at night?

When patients with insomnia come into the clinic, we always ask them right off the bat if they're napping, and if so, how long and how much. One of the *first* things we do for people with insomnia is ask them not to nap. If folks are having trouble falling asleep, the number-one thing they need to do is *keep* all of that sleep pressure they've been building up all day, and save it for bedtime. Think of a nap like this: it lets some of the air out of that sleep-pressure balloon. So yes, you may wake up feeling boosted and refreshed, but you'll also need to fill that balloon back up before you can fall asleep again.

With people who are struggling with sleep for whatever reason, the general recommendation is: don't nap. But if you *do* need to nap, keep it to twenty to thirty minutes, the magic length of a good nap. Why not longer? First, keeping it short makes sure that you're not "stealing" from nighttime sleep. And second, cutting it off at thirty minutes generally ensures that you won't dip into deep sleep, also known as N3 sleep.

Let's pause for one moment here to talk about *sleep architecture*—that's the term we use in sleep science to refer to the structure of your sleep.

## Your Sleep Blueprint

Your sleep has a blueprint and follows a predictable pattern: over the course of a night of sleep, you'll typically go through between four and six sleep cycles. Within each of those four cycles, you experience two types of sleep: non-REM (NREM) sleep, and REM sleep. REM stands for *rapid eye movement*. Not the most thrilling names, we know, but the reason we categorize sleep in this way is that these two different "types" of sleeping each fulfill very different functions.

**Non-REM (NREM) sleep comes first.** As you drop into sleep, you enter the first of three stages of NREM sleep, the N1 stage.

N1 stage sleep is light. Your sensory system isn't as lost to the world—you can still perceive sounds and stimuli around you, and you can easily be woken up. Next, you slip into the N2 stage.

N2 is characterized by what we call "sleep spindles": bursts of neural activity that occur as you're sleeping. Your brain, while you sleep, is actually very active. This is not downtime for your brain—it's just in a different mode. In N2, these neural bursts, which can be seen on an EEG, are indicative of brain activity tied to learning: we believe that this is where we are replaying, consolidating, and making new connections.

Finally, we get to N3. This stage is what we call *slow-wave sleep*. This is the deep, restorative sleep. It's also the phase that's hardest to wake from—if you're yanked out of slow-wave sleep, you're going to have a hard reentry.

**REM sleep comes last.** After you cycle through the three stages of non-REM sleep, you hit REM sleep, named so because of the eye movements that characterize this phase. This is where you do your dreaming. You are out of slow-wave sleep now; your sleep is lighter and you are closer to consciousness. But you are affected by muscle atonia—a kind of "sleep paralysis" that keeps you from getting out of bed and acting out your dreams.

The length of each phase of your sleep changes over the course of the night: in the early morning, close to the time you may be waking up, your non-REM sleep gets shorter, and your REM sleep goes on for longer. When you wake up naturally after completing a full sleep cycle, you may remember your dreams— that's because your sleep cycle (average length is about ninety minutes total) often ends with REM sleep. When you're waking up in the morning, you've most likely just been dreaming.

These cycles are dynamic, and they change from cycle to cycle as you progress through the night, and from person to person. We aren't robots. But we do know that if you're napping and you dip into slow-wave sleep, you're going to feel worse after—not better. When we wake up from a deep sleep, we're cognitively fuzzy and lethargic. That's called "sleep inertia." We don't always make it all the way into deep sleep within twenty to thirty minutes, but when sleep-deprived, we tend to drop into slow-wave sleep faster.

If you really need a nap, take a nap. Set an alarm for twenty minutes and go for it—you know your body, your sleep needs, and your schedule best. But honestly, if you came into my clinic and told me you were having trouble falling asleep, I'd tell you to skip it. I'd advise you to hoard that sleep pressure and save it for bedtime. I'd tell you to pour out that late-afternoon coffee or tea—and I'd pour mine out right along with you. Here's what I advise people to do instead.

## Boosting Yourself over the Afternoon Dip . . . Without Sabotaging Tonight

Your circadian rhythm might drag you down a bit in the afternoon—there's nothing you can do about that. And if you're having a tough time getting to sleep, staying asleep, or getting good-quality sleep, the sleep debt is going to be nipping at your heels right around then. So I want to take you through a couple of general strategies and mental shifts that can help you, and then we'll hop right into today's practice.

First: *optimize your schedule* today. Think about how you might structure your day to take better advantage of your peaks of alertness and to take the pressure off yourself during your circadian dip. When you can pinpoint your circadian highs of alertness and energy, you can plan your day to more effectively take advantage of them. Try to tackle the more cognitively demanding stuff during your natural energy highs. If you need to be creative and focused, to pay close attention or think deeply and brainstorm—ride those highs! Bump your busywork or other less-demanding tasks into those low-energy holes. Some circadian-savvy folks will even take a long break in the late afternoon, and return to urgent creative or strategic work in the early evening when they can ride that second energy high. (Just don't try to surf that wave right into bed—more on this later.)

Another strategy that works here is (don't hate me) **meditation**. We talked about meditation in the last chapter—mindfulness meditation in particular—as an effective tool for preventing stress buildup over the course of the day. I also mentioned that seasoned meditators seem somehow, strangely, to need less sleep than the average person—due, researchers think, to the way that brain states during meditation mimic slow-wave restorative sleep. So a short meditation session can be not only a stress-buster, but it can refresh you the way a short nap can. When we picture meditation, we might think of someone in a restful, slow, "paused" sort of state—but in fact meditation is quite mentally active, and can have an energizing effect on your system.

Next up: **move your body**. I'll admit it: this isn't the first thing I leap to when I need a pick me up. I'd much rather press the button on my Keurig and enjoy the toasty, bitter, delicious scent of hot coffee that's about to become liquid energy in my veins. But I've been swayed by the science. There's data showing that the effects of exercise on important cognitive processes, like working memory, are similar to the effects of caffeine.[5]

Next: **You don't need coffee to take a break**. Somehow it's easier to take a "coffee break" than it is to just take a break. But I think that much of the time, what the brain and body is really crying out for when it propels you toward the coffee machine or the corner cafe is other things: Movement. Fresh air. A change of scenery. If you're tired, restless, sluggish, and your mind is wandering, you might not need a jolt of caffeine—you might just need a quick switch-up from what you're doing. Try this: take a very short break—just five or ten minutes should do it—and just do something that you find enjoyable, and that's accessible and easy in your current environment. Some things people have told me they'll do: Walk around the block. Go out into the garden and pull weeds. Put on some music. Reorganize a bookshelf. When you come back to what you were doing before, I'm willing to bet you'll have a surge of energy and focus to help you out.

Anything that **switches up your routine** is going to help you out here. Break out of the mold of your typical day-to-day. Something new, different, or atypical is going to be arousing to the brain. Why? Because *novelty* inherently causes cognitive arousal. Quite literally, more of your neurons are firing. The arousal system whirrs to life and pushes a little more energy into your system via cortisol. Just mixing things up a little can naturally, effortlessly, and without the long dragging half-life of a stimulant, give you a little push to feel better and do better toward the end of your day.

And on that note, let's try out today's practice, which really capitalizes on the science of novelty and your arousal system.

TODAY'S PRACTICE

# STICK YOUR HEAD IN THE FREEZER

Yes! I mean it. Stick your head in the freezer: *it's science.*

A mild physical shock to the system might be exactly what you need today at 3 p.m. to beat that circadian dip you're feeling. We're not talking about anything extreme here—I'm not going to tell you to go take a cold shower or a polar bear swim. But the principle is the same: cold impacts the nervous system. If it's tamped down to a low idle and your energy has tanked, a brief cold exposure can act on you like jumper cables on a car battery.

In the lab, we use something called a "cold pressor task." For this condition, which we use to test people's physiological responses to various stressors, we put the participant's hand or forearm in ice-cold water. They have to keep it there for as long as they can stand it. Meanwhile, we're measuring their physiology with electrodes, tracking their heart rate and breathing. What we see is that it activates the cardiovascular system, leading to vasoconstriction (blood vessels shrink, slowing blood flow) and increased blood pressure. When your fight-or-flight system is engaged, you get an arousal response along with it. Now, with the cold pressor task, we're not sending people into fight-or-flight . . . but they are certainly experiencing systemic arousal. The sensation of bearing with the cold also presents an opportunity: to "train" yourself for stress resilience. What we know is that a little bit of physical stress can be good for you. We have growing evidence that intermittent stress exposure, known as *hormetic stress*, can give a positive boost to health and longevity.

Do you want to be in fight-or-flight mode? No. But *challenge stress* is great for your system. When you experience "peak and recovery" stress—where your acute stress response turns on, but then you recover quickly and your system goes back to baseline—it's actually healthy for your body at the cellular level . . . *and* it has an energizing effect. The key is to try to frame the stressor you're facing as a challenge to be overcome, rather than a threat to retreat from.

In my own life, I've found that stress can be an energizing force—as long as I'm able to view it as a challenge and not a threat. Here's my example: public speaking. I hate it! But I still do it. And at this point, I've come to enjoy it. Even as I'm standing in the wings, awash in stress hormones, nauseous, a little panicked, and wishing I'd never agreed to it, I'm already looking forward to the rush of energy I get once I've completed the dreaded task and walked off stage. My colleague Dr. Wendy Berry Mendes here at UCSF always uses the example of a lion chasing a gazelle to illustrate the distinction between challenge stress and threat stress. You can imagine it in your mind's eye: a gazelle running for its life across the African savannah, the lion just behind, only seconds away from a kill. Both are using metabolic resources, both are exerting high levels of energy, both are—in other words—stressed. But whereas the gazelle is experiencing threat stress, the lion is experiencing challenge stress. Challenge stress is what we're going for—be the lion, not the gazelle today. Follow the steps below:

- When that afternoon slump hits, go stick your head in the freezer! And hang out there for as long as you can. (Or, if you can, fill the kitchen sink with cold water—as cold as you can make it—and immerse your forearms to recreate our "cold pressor" task in your own home.)

- While you're experiencing the blast of cold, notice if it feels uncomfortable. But bear with it. Try to relax into it. Just try to exist with the intense sensation of cold. When you're done, your system will be revved up: heart rate a little higher, nervous system engaged, alertness up.

- Going forward: This is a small "stressor" to your system, not a big one. But as your day goes on, if you catch yourself experiencing a stress response to something that happens, try to reframe it as exciting instead of threatening. Stress researcher Dr. Elissa Epel suggests that positive stress, like exercise, cold exposure, or a feeling of "challenge" stress that you can quickly recover from (rather than "threat" stress, which tends to linger) can trigger *hormesis*, a cellular cleanup process that promotes healing and longevity.[6] It's not only good for your sleep tonight, it's good for your cells, too.

## DAY 4

# WORRY EARLY

HUMANS ARE COMPLEX CREATURES. ONE OF THE MANY THINGS THAT sets us apart from our fellow mammals in the animal kingdom is our capacity to *imagine*. Using just our thoughts, we can time-travel into the past or future, reliving or rewriting events that have already occurred, inventing various scenarios and filling them with vivid sensory detail. It's an amazing capacity we have. And it's at the root of a lot of our success as a species. But all wrapped up in that nice package of evolutionary advantages are some downsides: worry, anxiety, rumination. Because we're so great at these "virtual reality" simulations of the past and the possible future, we can easily get wrapped up in thought patterns that keep us focused on problems we have no capacity to change. We relive stressful or upsetting moments, and then feel the associated emotions. We drive up our own stress levels, for no reason at all, and with no associated benefit. We are really, really good at this. If humanity had a resume, this would be on our list of "Top Skills."

During a busy day, we can often move our thoughts away from worries, fears, and regrets pretty easily. Personally, when I'm racing from one thing to the next at the lab, going through study data and then taking a phone call, I don't have a lot of opportunities to sit with my thoughts. Urgent tasks-at-hand are always there, claiming my attention and mental bandwidth. But when we get in bed, in the dark, in the quiet, in our soft, comfortable beds, our thoughts can get very, very loud. And *rumination*—when you replay events from the past you wish had gone better, as opposed to *worry*, which is more future-focused—is, we believe, one of the major pathways that perpetuates insomnia.

We ran a study to test this. Just exactly *how* powerful a sleep-stopper was rumination? To figure it out, we set up an elaborate ruse. Basically, we were going to intentionally make people feel bad, and then watch what happened at night.[1]

## Rumination, the Sleep-Killer

Participants who volunteered for this study didn't have to haul down to the clinic—they could participate from the comfort and solitude of their own homes. In fact, we needed them to be at home and to participate remotely so that we could set up a rigged scenario where they'd experience social rejection, which is, frankly, a pretty quick route to negative feelings. Basically, we were going to intentionally make them feel bad. But the participants didn't know this. Here's what they knew: over the two nights of the study, they'd watch a video quietly on the first night, and interact virtually with other study participants on the second night. In both cases, their role in the study would happen about one hour before bedtime. All the participants wore a research-grade wrist device, known as an actigraph, to measure their sleep across the night.

We dropped off a laptop to each participant, preloaded with the software they'd need to use. The first night was simple: each person was asked to watch a video on the laptop, and then go to bed. This first night was the "control condition"—it established a baseline for what each participant's typical sleep and sleep routine (bedtime) probably looked like. The second night got a bit more interesting.

The participants were instructed to boot up their laptops for the study activity at the same time as the night before. But this time, the moderator asked them to log into Google Chat so they could interact with other study participants, who were also in their own homes, participating remotely. Except there *were* no "other study participants"—just my research assistant, moderating the study, and at the same time, controlling some avatars that *looked* like other study participants. Pre-study, each person had been asked to choose an emoji to represent themself. The fake study participants—called "confederates"— had emojis, too, and so on the second night of the study, two of these confederates entered the Google Chat with our real, actual participant.

Our actual participants, sitting at their laptops and believing they were chatting with other real live humans, were asked to play a simple game called "cyberball" with their new virtual acquaintances. This was decidedly not a high-tech virtual reality experience—just a basic pixelated game. There's a ball, and you choose whom to throw it to. You can throw to one person, then the other. This little blinking ball is tossed from player to player, from one emoji-avatar to the other. It's such a simple, largely pointless game that pretty quickly, people are probably wondering what the point of it is. But then, at a certain point, the two confederates, controlled by the moderator, cut the study participant out of the game. Now, the real person is watching these two play the game.

This scenario has been run before in scientific studies—we didn't invent this. It's known to produce feelings of ostracism and social rejection. One frequently cited paper[2] had study participants play the game while *inside an MRI scanner,* and the scans showed that the rejection people experienced during the exclusion part of the game activated the canonical pain regions of the brain. It literally caused social pain. So, we know that this exercise is a fairly reliable way to get a study participant into this particular headspace, to then test out what kind of impact it has on various other factors. But it's also pretty mild. We wanted to up the ante a bit. So at this point, the moderator cuts in with some news for our real live human participant: "You've been randomly selected to give a speech!"

The participant is given a topic that they need to immediately expound upon; the confederates are asked to give feedback in the chat. The pressure is *on.* Topics we've used: *What makes you a good friend? Do you support how Walmart treats its employees? What do you think about Google controlling so much of the internet's ad revenue?*

Our participant turns on their video and begins to speak; the confederates start offering their observations:

"You sound kind of nervous."

"What you just said doesn't actually make that much sense."

"Wow I'm so glad I didn't have to do this, this is kind of rough!"

Eventually, the confederates pivot to talking to each other about something completely off-topic. The participant can see the chat and realizes that the other "people" in the study aren't paying any attention.

Finally, the moderator wraps it all up.

"OK, thank you for participating!" he says into the speaker. "Good night!"

People's initial reactions to experiencing all this varied. Some people forged ahead with their speech, a little annoyed. Some got rattled. One person got so upset, she just slammed the laptop shut, cutting the whole thing short. Our prediction was, obviously, that people would sleep less after having this experience. And in fact, they did. But there were some interesting nuances within the data. The people who participated stayed up *way* later than they had on their control night. It wasn't that they got into bed at their usual time and then couldn't fall asleep—they just stayed up, presumably because they had so much arousal surrounding the stressful incident. Also, prior to the study, we'd had them fill out a rumination questionnaire that assessed their tendency toward rumination in general, on a sliding scale, from low to high. It turned out that the biggest difference surrounding sleep after this incident of social rejection occurred in the *high rumination* people. People who were low on the rumination scale were much less affected.

So what does this tell us? That the more you tend toward high rumination, the more affected you're going to be by events in the day you perceive as negative, stressful, or threatening. Even ambiguous or neutral events can be viewed through a more negative lens by high ruminators. What people end up with is a state of constant arousal that really does get in the way of their capacity to transition themselves to bedtime and fall asleep. Sleep requires letting go of that level of vigilance; rumination causes us to remain vigilant and on high alert, replaying the events of the day, the past week, or the past years over and over in our minds. They are completely incompatible mental processes.

## How Prone to Rumination Are *You*?

The takeaway from this study was that if you tend toward rumination in general, you're going to be more affected by "regrettable events" in your day. Social rejection was really effective at disturbing people's sleep, but other regrettable events can be similarly potent. We zeroed in on social rejection in this instance because in humans, who are by nature pack animals, it causes a strong and reliable negative reaction. We're social by nature—even the introverts—and we're very sensitive and susceptible to interpersonal slights. A good example of how powerful this is: interpersonal stressors like a romantic breakup are one of the strongest predictors of a depressive episode, compared to other major stressors or life disruptions people might experience.[3] A feeling of being "less than" can actually translate to tangible effects on physical health. In scientific studies like this one, we routinely use things that have social evaluation as part of it, whether explicit or implicit, because we are able to clearly measure impact: we see effects reflected in the stress system[4]—higher cortisol in the bloodstream, greater sympathetic nervous system activity, impaired cognitive processes—and we see effects on sleep.

In this study, the negative experience caused people to lose, on average, an hour of sleep. The closer to bedtime, the bigger the impact (less time to process and move past it). And the more prone to rumination people were, the bigger the impact.[5]

Why are some people naturally more ruminative than others? There's a whole cornucopia of factors. Brain chemistry is partially genetic—we are simply born with certain tendencies. We also know that adversity early in life can lead to a tendency to ruminate more, in part because people who've gone through hardship may be more on alert and perceive innocuous stimuli as negative or threatening, which may in turn trigger a stress response that includes rumination. And finally, certain mental patterns become ingrained the more we do them. Neural pathways are like paths in the forest; the more we tread them, the more established and permanent they become. But there's good news within that metaphor: just like a forest path, they can fade with less use. The human brain has incredible neuroplasticity.

The brain, this central command center for our behaviors and personalities, our habits and beliefs, can be literally reshaped. In other words, if you are a high ruminator, you are not doomed. It can change. But let's figure out, roughly, where your starting point is:

- Is your attention often focused on aspects of yourself you wish you could stop thinking about?
- Do you find it hard to shut off thoughts about yourself?
- Do you often waste time rethinking things that are over and done with?
- Do you have a tendency to dwell on yourself for too long?
- Do you often reflect on episodes of your life that you should no longer concern yourself with?

If you've answered yes to all of these questions, you're likely someone who is more prone to rumination. Rumination is normal. It's a totally natural human compulsion. We believe that we can solve these problems that haunt us if we just think them through—the trouble is, so many of the problems we try to solve (while lying in the dark at night) are not solvable. They are perpetual problems—problems of being human. Our minds return to them incessantly, convinced that we can puzzle them out like algebra. We can't, but we keep trying.

Unsurprisingly, worry and rumination went *way* up during COVID. The waiting list for our sleep clinic became pages and pages long. Surveys showed that more people reported insomnia. Anxiety, depression, worry—it all went through the roof during COVID, especially early on.[6] People were reporting more difficulty falling asleep and *staying* asleep—there was a spike in early morning wake ups. People would pop awake at 4 a.m. and then not be able to fall back asleep, which makes sense: sleep gets lighter in the early morning hours, so a likely cause is that if you have stressors on board, they're much more likely to jolt you awake during that pre-dawn stretch of lighter REM sleep. Plus, our media consumption was up as much as 60 percent according to Nielsen,[7] which tracks television and media usage. Media consumption, especially during times of collective stress or trauma, is the enemy of sleep. It's a constant stream of content that is terrible and worrisome, fed right into that virtual reality simulator inside your skull. If you had even a little bit of a tendency toward rumination, the worldwide, never-before-in-our-lifetime events we all experienced certainly provided ample fodder for "dark night of the soul" mental spinning. It's a vicious cycle: rumination makes it more difficult to sleep well, and when you don't get the sleep you need, you're more vulnerable to rumination. Your ability to stave off intrusive thoughts weakens and falters. Your mental armor is brittle.

Personally, I'm not much of a ruminator, and yet it still gets me sometimes. Anybody is vulnerable to the agitating thought-loops of rumination, given the right triggers, pressures, or stressors. And rumination can lead to a prolonged stress response. So aside from practicing radical acceptance like a Buddhist monk, what do we *do*?

I could get all Zen on you here and tell you that what you really need to do is learn to accept these conflicts and discomforts as part of the human condition—but I'm not going to.

## Getting off the Rumination Track

The best in-the-moment fix for rumination is cutting right to the root cause of why rumination is such a sleep-blocker: it keeps your mind aroused. Your attention is drawn back, again and again, to this thing that didn't go well, to a mistake or a regret. I've laid in bed and replayed a dumb thing I said at a party—something the person I said it to probably forgot about moments later, but which my dogged mind clings to. It's easy to spiral from something small like that to sweeping generalizations about yourself and the mistakes you *always* make. Negative thoughts and emotions like these are what neuroscientists call "salient": they are very *loud*. Like a shout or a car horn, they grab our attention effortlessly. And negative content is hard to look away from.

One memorable patient of mine at the sleep clinic had a particular struggle with this. When I met Myra, she'd been sent to me from a special neurology unit. She was young, in her early thirties, and newly married. Everybody at the clinic loved her—she was outgoing, upbeat, always happy. She came in and lit up the room. She also had a fairly severe form of epilepsy. She had seizures constantly—I realized later that she'd have multiple seizures during our sessions, when we were in the middle of conversation. To me, it just looked like she was distracted, or taking a minute to gather her thoughts. She'd learned to cope and cover, saying, "Where were we?" or "Just lost my train of thought for a minute there . . ." But the seizures were serious and limiting. She'd already had one surgical brain resection in an effort to stop the seizures from happening. In this type of brain surgery, called a temporal lobectomy, neurosurgeons will actually remove a section of the brain that's causing the seizures. (The fact that people can and do go on to recover from these surgeries is another great argument for brain neuroplasticity!) Myra's epilepsy, however, was unfortunately still so severe, it was looking like they'd need to perform another brain resection to try to get it under control. There was just one last thing to try before resorting to invasive brain surgery again that they thought might help: *sleep*.

As with a lot of chronic illnesses, sleep can play a role in epilepsy symptoms. Lack of sleep is known to trigger seizures, and Myra's sleep was not great. She was spending a ton of time in bed awake, trying to fall asleep. She had an enormous amount of anxiety surrounding her ability to sleep—understandable, since in her case, poor sleep really did have immediate health consequences for her, leaving her struggling with depression and more vulnerable to seizures, more fatigued, and less able to do the things she wanted to do during the day. A result of all this was that she spent a lot of time lying in bed with her mind spinning. She described not being able to stop thinking. She would worry about tomorrow; she would ruminate on things she should have done differently today. All kinds of negative, distracting thoughts would pop into her mind.

Myra's specific struggle with epilepsy might have been unique to her, but her tendency to be kept awake by her own thoughts was not. Many—if not most—people I see in the clinic struggle with this to some extent. I suggested she try a tactic that works for most people: "cloud watching," where you imagine those unwanted thoughts as clouds, gliding by overhead and passing out of sight. It's a fairly standard tactic that draws on tenets of mindfulness meditation, specifically, *open monitoring*, which trains practitioners to allow thoughts to "pass through" their minds. Instead of engaging with the content that the mind produces, one maintains a kind of distance, letting thoughts simply fade—or drift out of sight like a cloud scudding across the sky.

Myra laughed and tilted her head curiously. "Who watches *clouds*?" she wanted to know.

The whole idea was bizarre and hilarious to her—she had never laid on her back in the grass watching a cloud, and didn't get why anyone would. It made sense that the exercise wouldn't resonate with her, now that I thought about it—she was a *go go go* type of person, always in motion, always with a meticulously organized to-do list as long as her arm.

But there was another way to get at the same concept, maybe even a better way, that more accurately reflected the way intrusive and ruminative thoughts work in the human brain. I thought of an article I'd been reading recently about a practice in Europe called *trainspotting*. Some may know it as a dark and gritty movie from the 1990s; it's also a niche hobby among certain railway enthusiasts, who like to collect train sightings the way birdwatchers collect species. They hang out on train platforms waiting for what they call "rolling stock" to go by, then try to snap a picture or note the make and model. One thing they do not do is get *on* the train. They just watch it blow by.

"So when you have these thoughts when you're trying to fall asleep, you can either be on the train, or you can be on the platform," I told Myra. "If you're on the train, you're along for the ride. You get whisked off to wherever, and you're totally immersed—you see everything the train goes through, and it's all really stimulating. But those trains are going to destinations that are not helpful."

Instead, stay on the platform. The train comes through, but you don't get on. You notice it—you can't help but notice it—but you don't go with it. You check it out and let it go by.

Trainspotting worked a lot better than cloud watching for Myra. It made more intuitive sense—for her, it was easy to be mentally transported somewhere that was stressful, or sad, or worrying, and not good at all for sleep. It was hard not to metaphorically get on the train: those thoughts that arrived came roaring in like a train with a whistle. They weren't soft and fluffy like clouds, gently passing by. They were loud, intrusive, and demanding of her attention. But when she thought of herself as a "thought spotter," she was able to put some distance between herself and the ruminative mental content keeping her awake.

## When Your Own Mind Is the Problem

Sleep, it seems, should be so easy. It's natural. It's necessary. Our bodies need it, literally, to stay alive. It's as essential as food, water, and oxygen. And yet all of these conditions of living, of being human, conspire to get in our way—our own minds in particular. The contents of our ruminations and our worries do not appear out of nowhere. We pull from the world around us and from our pasts. The experiences we have throughout our days are the raw content for the mental chatter we may experience at night, chatter that can lead to hypervigilance: an inability to feel safe and let go. Any of us can end up having daily experiences that wind up on our minds, but the truth is that exposure to things that cause the kind of stress, worry, and rumination that disrupt sleep are not evenly distributed across the population. We know, for instance, that in the United States, Black Americans experience higher rates of chronic stress exposures than white Americans, and have poorer health outcomes linked to the wear and tear of long-term activation of the stress-response system.[8] This has profound implications for sleep disparities.

In a study that we're running now, supported by the National Institute of Health, we're taking that scenario from the beginning of the chapter—with social rejection—but tweaking it slightly by changing the race of the emojis. For example, some of our Black participants will be randomized to receive social rejection from emojis that look like a white participant while others will receive rejection from an emoji that represents a

Black participant. The same will be true for our white participants. What we hope to learn, among other things, is how much
does the experience of discrimination affect our sleep physiology? As we continue to uncover the deep and long-lasting health
impacts of racial discrimination, this is a critical factor to nail
down. Sleep, after all, is the foundation that so much of our physical and mental health is built upon. A study on first-generation
Latinx college students discovered that the more discrimination these students experienced, the more their sleep worsened
over the course of the school year.[9] While we certainly need to
gather additional hard data, there's reason to believe that cognitive processes, like rumination, are key mechanisms through
which adverse experiences like racism and discrimination sabotage sleep.

In the clinic, I work with people who face all kinds of obstacles to sleep that are completely beyond their control. They live
somewhere with a lot of nighttime noise and can't afford to
move. They are affected by domestic violence. They don't feel
secure where they live. One young artist I worked with described living below a loud neighbor in his thin-walled apartment in Oakland: almost every night, there was intermittent
shouting and fighting. Even in the periods of silence, he said, he
would be anxious about when the *next* sound might arrive, and
the anticipation would keep him awake. We tried all kinds of
tactics, but there's not much that can help in this kind of situation outside of moving, which was not an option for him, or, I
guess, a *really* good pair of earplugs. When he stopped coming
into the clinic, I wondered what had happened—had he figured

out some ingenious way to create an impenetrable mental shield, like a Zen master, to block out the intrusive noises once and for all? So often, when people disappear from the sleep clinic, we aren't sure why—did they get better? Did they get frustrated and give up? I reached out to him to find out.

"Oh," he said, "the guy moved away!"

We both laughed. But then he went on to tell me that the issue hadn't actually vanished with the noisy neighbor. Now, it was quiet at night. But he had the same low-level anxiety that something was going to wake him up just as he was falling asleep. And that something was usually his own brain.

"It just feels like my mind is so good at coming up with something that *really* bothers me right when I lay down to sleep," he said. "It's just as disturbing as the yelling next door used to be. Now it's just . . . in my head."

Not all of the factors that impact our sleep are within our control. But our own minds—loud and persistent as they can be—can indeed be managed. There are things we can do, proactively, to set ourselves up for a more peaceful night inside our own heads.

TODAY'S PRACTICE

# PUT IT IN THE PARKING LOT

The best time to get ahead of worry and rumination is during the day, before the sun even starts to set. There's no magical switch to completely turn off rumination—you have a human brain, and part of its job is to consolidate information and build new synapses by dredging up moments from your day, memories from the past, stuff that upset you, and so forth. Your brain has a pretty good reason for doing most of what it does—it just gets off track. Today, so that you don't get caught up in ruminative loops that keep your cortisol up and your brain active and awake, we're going to swipe some of that rumination fodder off your plate before bedtime even hits.

I want to offer you two choices of practices: pick one, or try both. Both of them are going to help you to do what I call "putting it in the parking lot." It basically means setting unfinished business to the side and not letting it follow you home and into bed.

## Strategy #1: Worry Early

Today, and for the rest of this week, set aside a specific chunk of time for something very important to your well-being. It's not a massage or a hot bath. It's not me-time—though if you're following yesterday's instruction to take a break, you hopefully got some of that as well! This is time exclusively for *worrying*. Yes: today, you're going to worry on purpose.

I recommend choosing a time during the mid- to late-afternoon because it's early enough that it won't impact your ability to go to sleep later, but it's not so early that you still have a big chunk of your day left to go to produce rumination-creating foibles.

Set a timer for fifteen minutes. This is your daily, intentional worry time. Don't do anything else while you do this—it defeats the purpose. If possible, go someplace where you can be uninterrupted. Some of my patients have locked themselves in the bathroom to avoid being disturbed. Some people take a walk. Do what you need to do!

Once that timer starts, you are going to give yourself the freedom to worry. Worry about one topic at a time. Think of it like a to-do list that you go through one by one, except what you're checking off are the topics you feel the most anxiety about during the day (and then night), the ones your mind returns to over and over, the topics that occupy all your mental space. You may spend a lot of time trying to stop yourself from thinking about this stuff too much—in this fifteen-minute window, just let yourself go. One important caveat: this is not problem-solving time. The expectation is *not* that you come out of this with everything solved. Your entire goal is *just to worry*, fruitlessly, obsessively.

You can write it all down in a journal, say it out loud to a nearby tree, dictate a recording onto your phone—or just think about it. It's important to spend this focused attention on it. When that timer goes off after fifteen minutes, though, you're done.

If you notice during the day that you find yourself worrying, you can say to yourself, *Look, you need to just postpone this to the next worry time. You have time set aside for this. It can wait until tomorrow—you have it scheduled.* Use this exact same technique if worries are popping up again at bedtime: *You have this scheduled for tomorrow.* If you find yourself gripped by that worry anyway, write it down. Tonight, before bed, make sure you have paper and pen nearby. If a worry or anxious thought shows up, write it down, so you can remember to focus on it at your next scheduled worry time. If you like, you can thank your worries for stopping by and tell them you'll see them tomorrow. (I'd recommend projecting that thought in a spirit of goodwill rather than passive aggression, but to each their own.)

One final note: There's nothing special about fifteen minutes. It could be ten or twenty—do what works for you. Keep in mind though that we want it to be enough time that you can be present and get some of this worry off your plate. Do this daily for the rest of the week and see how it works for you. Hopefully it will lead to reduced worrying and rumination at nighttime, which is going to help your "conditioned response" to the bedroom—which we'll build upon in the next chapter.

## Strategy #2: Constructive Worry

On a piece of paper, create two columns, the first labeled "Problem" and the other labeled "Solution." Come up with a short list of current problems that you're dealing with. Focus in particular on topics you're likely to ruminate over tonight. Then, come up with the next one to three steps you could take to tackle each issue—place these on the solution side. Basically, you're charting out a plan for how to get started on addressing each problem.

Note: you're not making a plan for how to solve the problem completely; nor are you actually solving it right now. This is your blueprint for how to get started—actionable steps that are doable tomorrow, or at least within the next few days.

Now, take the paper and fold it up. As soon as you're able, put it right by your bed and say to yourself, "I have come up with a plan for these things for when I'm at my best, sharper than I am in the middle of the night. I can wait to do these things until tomorrow because I have a plan." It may sound silly, but there really is something to this ritual: bearing witness to the fact that you already spent focused energy on these problems, so can now release your mind from the purgatory of puzzling over them interminably during the night.

If any of this stuff pops up for you at bedtime, just remind yourself: "I have a plan." Some people I've worked with will even reach out and touch the paper.

This technique may be especially helpful if you're prone

to waking up in the middle of the night to worry. How often have you tried to solve things in the middle of the night, then you wake up in the morning and have no idea what the solution was? Late at night, we're not cognitively there. Three in the morning is *not* the time to figure out your financial problems or how to handle a conflict with your spouse. You're wasting your time, and you're shorting yourself on sleep. You'll be in a much better place the next day if you *don't* do this, and instead wait until the next day when you have the energy and the cognitive capacity.

## Troubleshooting

With patients affected by nighttime rumination and worry, I really do see that prevention makes a huge difference for them. And that's why this proactive approach is what I'm asking you to try today, and to add to your routine for the rest of this week (and hopefully longer, if this works for you). But often there are things that surface in the moment that you wouldn't have anticipated: deeper worries, or topics that surprise you. Like a scary movie where you've prepared yourself for one type of monster, and what pops out of the closet is something else entirely.

In this case, there's a couple things you can try. One is the "trainspotting" exercise I described earlier in this chapter: picture yourself on that platform, watching the thoughts arrive and depart, arrive and depart.

Or, when all else fails? *Distraction.* Think about something else.

Sound too simple? Well, it might be but it's also science. When you do it right, distraction can be a powerful sleep aid to squash rumination. Here's the reason it works: your working memory, which is where you basically do all your thinking, planning, imagining, and ruminating, is only so large. It has limits. You can't think about ten things at once. Neuroscientists have discovered that the number of discrete things you can think about at once is about three. After that, stuff just blips off your radar. If you've ever walked into a room and had no idea why you were there, you know exactly what I mean—it happened because you started thinking about something else, and one balloon bopped the other one right into the stratosphere.

So here, I'm just asking you to do that on purpose. If you're awake, thinking about stuff you don't want to be thinking about, fill up your mind with another balloon. The catch is, it has to be something good. Sleep-medicine experts will often help people come up with vivid, engaging imagery: places they can go in their mind that are pleasant or soothing to them.

To use visualization to replace negative thought loops, try this:

- Start with progressive muscle relaxation. Lie on your back in bed and begin at the top of your head and slowly move down the body, going muscle by muscle, as precisely as you can, until you reach your toes. Tense each muscle, then release. Move to the next area. Tense and then release. Let the weight of your physical body press down into the bed. Then . . .

- Visualize a place that's serene for *you* (sitting on the beach, on a grassy hill on a sunny day, being by a lake, walking through the woods hearing a river). It can be a real place you know from memory, or an invented place.
- Focus on the sensory details of this place—the sounds, the smells, what you touch and feel. Move your mind from one sensation to the next: The sound of the waves. The warmth of the sand under your hands. The smell of pine trees and the spongy feeling of dirt under your feet as you walk through the forest. Whatever place you pick, illustrate it with the five senses as richly as possible.

Doing this takes cognitive effort and uses up your cognitive bandwidth. It's simple: it's incompatible with rumination. And focusing on sensory details to recreate the experience leaves little space for your mind to be on those negative, ruminative thoughts.

## DAY 5

# YOU ARE NOT A COMPUTER, YOU CAN'T JUST SHUT DOWN

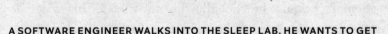

**A SOFTWARE ENGINEER WALKS INTO THE SLEEP LAB. HE WANTS TO GET** off the sleep meds he's been taking—he and his doctors feel he's become too dependent on them. His goal in visiting us is to learn to fall asleep on his own. Meanwhile, he tells us, he is pursuing a master's degree in computer programming and studies right up until bedtime. He's a busy man! He needs to use every minute wisely. So, he works until midnight, takes his two sleep aids, shuts down his computer, then gets in bed and waits for his brain to shut down as well. And . . . it doesn't.

It usually takes until at least 1 a.m. for him to fall asleep, he tells me, even with the help of one of the sleep-inducing "Z-drugs" (zolpidem, eszopiclone, zaleplon) that are commonplace among those suffering from insomnia. Sometimes it takes longer. And he has to be up early to drive his wife to her early shift at a local eatery at 7:30 a.m. So if he doesn't fall asleep fast enough at night, he has to take a nap the next morning. Sometimes he feels so tired and is so worried about how little sleep he got, that he takes a nap in the car in the parking lot at his wife's workplace.

So, we process this guy—his name's Omar—into the clinic as an insomnia case. Omar tells us he's tired but having trouble falling asleep at night. He feels so strongly about needing more sleep and is so fearful about dozing off while driving that he'll sleep in the car in a parking lot. Yet at the same time, he's not actually prioritizing sleep at all. He's working intensively right up until he wants to be asleep, then depending on medicinal sleep aids to get him there. But even that's not working so well anymore, because he's not allowing any time for his system to transition into sleep. He's expecting an immediate shutoff.

Right off the bat, it's pretty clear what the problem is—and it's probably clear to you, too. But at the same time, just being able to identify this problem doesn't mean we can easily solve it. We live in an on-demand culture where sleep becomes the last thing on our list to check off—the last thing we do when everything else in our day is completed. And yet, sleep is the thing that unlocks our capacity to do what we want to do, be who we want to be. We know this, but the pressure we get from the culture to be busy and productive is real. A lot of people have trouble justifying taking the time they need for sleep—and for easing into sleep—and end up turning to quicker strategies (medications) or having unrealistic expectations of how sleep should happen, like Omar.

To start the process of weaning him off his sleep medications to allow him to fall asleep naturally, I told him that to begin, he'd need to stop working no later than 11 p.m., take his medications, and then wind down for an hour. Then he might actually be able to fall asleep around midnight and achieve his goal of six and a half hours.

"Hmm," he said, clearly not into the idea. "What if I take my meds at eleven, but keep working until midnight . . ."

"Look, man," I said, "you work with computers. But you're not a computer. You can't just turn your brain off and go to sleep like that."

What he really wanted was to game the system. He wanted there to be a way to "optimize" all of his time awake, right up until he got in bed and powered down. And he wanted that power-down to happen immediately. But his *goal* in coming to work with us was to get off his sleep meds. And these two objectives were entirely incompatible.

What we needed to work on with him—and quite honestly, with the vast majority of people who come into the clinic with sleep struggles—was creating the time and ritual necessary for him to go to sleep naturally, in a way that worked within the context of his life.

## You Can't Game the System

Of the people who arrive at our clinic, 90 percent are on some type of sleep medication. You might be on one. Some take them when they travel, or when they really need to make sure they get a good night's sleep because there's something that requires their full attention the next day. Sleep aids can be a helpful and necessary intervention, but like any medication, there are side effects and risk factors associated with long-term use. A lot of people come to us because their medication use has gone beyond the occasional, emergency use. Many begin to fear that they can't sleep without medications. Often they've tried to quit, gone cold turkey, and then experienced a really bad night of sleep, called *rebound insomnia*. This sends people right back into the arms of their meds, resigned to taking a pill to ensure they get enough sleep to function. So, when patients arrive at our clinic, they show up with the goal of not only improving their sleep, but unhooking from their dependence on pharmaceutical sleep aids.

When it comes to falling asleep at night, we have a lot working against us. We live in a busy culture. We value performance and productivity over health and well-being—often ignoring the fact that those two things are, in fact, deeply linked. We feel guilty for taking time to relax, and so we de-prioritize rest. We have an entrenched belief that our time awake should be "used" productively. We understand that sleep is essential for our health in the long term, yet we de-prioritize it in the short term, day after day. We expect that if we're tired enough, sleep will just happen. We expect to be able to think ourselves to sleep, or will ourselves to sleep.

But we also have a lot working *for* us. Powerful biological forces are at work twenty-four hours a day: circadian rhythm is pushing us toward sleep. Our homeostatic sleep drive, that sleep "pressure" that's been building up all day, is pressing on us. All the various zeitgebers throughout the day, like when we eat or exercise, go to work and come home, are all being gathered up by our body, data points that assist with the dispensing of cortisol or melatonin and rising adenosine, the hormones that either keep us alert or lull us toward sleep. These are all happening, no matter what else we're doing. So a lot of the time, what we really need is to learn how to get out of our own way. And that means setting aside, and then ferociously protecting, the time it takes to transition from *awake* to *asleep*.

## How to Fall Asleep: Flipping the Switch

You get sleepy. You lie down in bed. And at some point, you sink into sleep, like dropping under the surface of some warm, soothing water. It feels gradual. But when we examine what's happening on a neurological level, it's a very different experience. In reality, when you drift off to sleep, it's like you're stepping off a cliff. But then you're transported back on top of the cliff. Then you fall off the "sleep cliff" again. Basically, there's a period of time where you go in and out of sleep. You can't be awake and asleep at the same time; there's no such thing as "half asleep." It's either/or. In neuroscience, they call it the "flip-flop switch."

There's a delicate balance between your arousal system and your sleep system. Both are neurochemical systems in the brain: they each have a network of neurons associated with them. On the wake side of the equation, we have wake-promoting neurons in the brain stem and hypothalamus and elsewhere that release histamine, dopamine, serotonin, and norepinephrine. On the sleep side, we have neurons in the ventrolateral preoptic nucleus of the hypothalamus that release GABA (and galanin). GABA may sound familiar, as GABA receptors are the primary targets for things like alcohol and antianxiety medications. These two systems are what we call "reciprocally inhibitory." In other words, when one is active, the other one is suppressed. At the moment of "falling asleep," what you're actually feeling is these two systems battling each other. An example where this switch seems to be broken is seen in people with narcolepsy. This is a condition where patients experience often overwhelming daytime sleepiness and suffer "attacks" of sleep. These sleep attacks tend to happen without warning and are associated with a complete loss of muscle tone, called cataplexy. The science is still developing but many of these patients lack sufficient hypocretin/orexin neurons, which are wake-promoting by nature and serve as a figurative referee in the battle between these wake- and sleep-promoting neurochemical systems.

The sleeping brain is incredibly complex. However, for our purposes, what finally tips the balance are those two sleep processes we've been talking about: homeostatic sleep drive and circadian rhythm. If your sleep pressure has built up enough (that balloon is nice and full) and your circadian rhythm is nicely aligned, you'll finally flip over to *asleep* and stay there.

One of the ways this happens is through the production of *melatonin*, often called the "sleep hormone."

Melatonin is a natural hormone produced by the pineal gland, which looks like a tiny pinecone (that's where the name comes from) and sits deep in your brain. Another hormone produced primarily in the raphe nucleus of the brain is *serotonin*, which is sometimes called the body's natural happiness hormone. The balance between the two hormones is one of the many moving pieces in this ongoing cycle that helps you fall asleep and wake up again, every day. And both are regulated, to a certain extent, by *light*. When you open the blinds in the morning and a blast of daylight hits your retina, the cells of the retina zing a signal back to the suprachiasmatic nucleus, where your "internal clock" lives. It, in turn, pings the pineal gland to stop melatonin, and at the same time leads to an increase in serotonin secretion. At night, the reverse happens: your retinal cells process the dimming of the natural light in your environment, and your pineal gland is notified to get that melatonin pumping.

Melatonin doesn't put you to sleep all on its own. It's not an Ambien! But it is certainly a critical piece of the going-to-sleep puzzle. For instance, at least in mice, melatonin inhibits wake-promoting hypocretin/orexin neurons, thus leading to sleep.[1] Along with adenosine, the presence of melatonin in the brain allows us to let go and succumb to sleep. Picture that flip-flop switch we were just talking about. Melatonin is like a thumb, pressing down on the *sleep* side. So the thing to consider is that the stuff you do in the hours before bed can either aid in melatonin production or get in its way.

## Making Melatonin

We don't go to bed with the sun anymore—it's been a long time since that's been a realistic thing for humans. We are bathed in artificial light, often right up until we go to sleep. It's a common piece of advice from sleep experts that you should start to knock down the decibel level of your light exposure a couple hours before bed. You've also probably heard a lot of advice to limit television, computer, and smartphone use before bed, because of the *type* of light these devices emit: blue light. Blue light, which has a shorter wavelength, has more of an impact on circadian processes. Research shows that it can suppress the production of melatonin like sunlight does. So basically you can think about it this way: if you're gazing into your phone at night, whether you're working on an email or relaxing by watching a show, it's a bit like gazing into a beam of sunlight.[2] The message your brain's getting is, *Wake up!*

If you Google "sleep hygiene," you're going to find a million articles telling you not to have any blue light exposure two hours before bed: no TV, no phone, no computer. And look— they're not wrong. Melatonin is a significant player in the onset of sleep, so you do want to be aware of that and limit your light exposure to the extent that you can. But this isn't an all-or-nothing situation. You don't have to sit in a pitch-black room listening to ocean sounds in order to prepare your brain and body to fall asleep. Limiting light exposure in the lead-up to bedtime *is* a good idea. It's one of the many levers you adjust and move to a setting that works for you. But I'm of the opinion that the blue-light exposure alone is not going to make or break your sleep success.

From where I sit, of all the things that impact people's sleep, the blue-light issue is probably a fairly minor one for most people. The industry that's cropped up around limiting blue light to preserve the melatonin system might be bigger than the actual problem. I went to my ophthalmologist recently and they wanted to put a purple tint on my lenses: "It's blue-light blocking, it'll help you sleep better!" they said. I said no, thanks. And they did it anyway.

I'm a sleep scientist—I know exactly what's happening when I lie in bed in the dark, scrolling through Twitter, and yet I still do it. I'm just as susceptible as anyone to the stimulus-reward loop of social media and phone apps. Sometimes what you're doing on your blue-light emitting device *is* actually relaxing—I always tell people it's OK to watch TV at night, for example. Sleep-advice websites tend to take a hard line on this and say "no screens," but look: not everybody is going to find relief from sitting in a chair and meditating. For some, that kind of thing amps up their anxiety when they become *more* aware of upsetting thoughts. Maybe what they really need is to softly zone out to reruns of *The Office* or *Sex and the City* (or whatever floats your boat). But a lot of the other stuff we do on our laptops, tablets, and phones does become way more of a problem—but it's not solely because of the blue light. It's that we become too engaged in them. The reward system in your brain is activated by the design of social-media apps. And what it wants most is . . . *more*.

That's what's keeping you awake. The light isn't helping, to be sure. But even if you get the purple tint on your glasses, if you're reading one stressful news story after another on your laptop before bed, you're still not going to be able to fall asleep. A blue-light filter isn't a magic bullet. The recommendation to disengage from your phone and other devices is an important one—but let's be clear about the reason. We can't engage in content that's going to get our nervous system fired up, no matter what type of light filter we use. It's not the light you need to turn off—it's the *engagement*.

## But What About Supplements?

Sleep supplements fill grocery-store shelves—not only melatonin, but other non-prescription sleep aids ranging from magnesium to valerian root to lavender elixirs. You can get them in pill form or gummy form. You can buy them for your kids. You can order them on Amazon.

My colleagues and I field endless questions about the efficacy of sleep aids. But the sleep aids we are asked about more than any others are related to marijuana. This probably isn't surprising to you. Across the United States, states are legalizing marijuana, and its active ingredient THC, for recreational use. In many cases marijuana can help with sleep, though this varies by strain. For example, sativa strains tend to make people feel energized while indica strains often produce feelings of relaxation, lethargy, and sleepiness. But what do we really know about THC or CBD and its efficacy to improve sleep problems? Unfortunately, not a lot. A couple of small randomized controlled trials testing cannabinoid formulations, which include THC and CBD, suggest that these ingredients can be helpful for improving sleep compared to placebo.[3] However, these studies are small and they evaluate formulations that are not readily available to people out in the world. The hope is that more research will be conducted in this area, because at present we are sort of flying blind.

One of the biggest issues with sleep supplements is the placebo effect: they may simply work because you believe they'll work. Dr. Alia Crum, a researcher at Stanford University who's done deep dives into placebo, calls this the "self-fulfilling prophecy": in short, you take a pill or supplement expecting it to help you sleep, and you're able to relax into sleep.

Nevertheless, synthetic melatonin (as opposed to *endogenous melatonin*, which is the natural hormone produced in your brain) is, in fact, the single most-used supplement by both adults and children in the United States. When it comes to our cultural struggle to fall asleep melatonin gets a lot of attention. Does it work?

Sure, melatonin supplements can help. They're especially effective for recovering from jet lag, or when we need to quickly shift someone's circadian clock, but less so for insomnia. However, if people come into the sleep clinic and are taking melatonin and report that it's working for them, I wouldn't tell them to stop, at least not at first. In the clinic, we've definitely heard from patients that supplementary melatonin can help to bring on sleepiness. But interestingly, when we taper people *off* the supplement, it doesn't typically make a difference for their sleep. They often don't notice the waning dosage, and then sleep just as well once they've phased it out completely.

The good news is that lack of THC or melatonin or whatever supplement you are taking is not the reason you are having sleep problems. In fact, one huge reason people have sleep problems has to do with the *expectation* of what it means to fall asleep. Going to sleep means letting go. It can be hard to make that transition, especially when you're holding onto vigilance from the day. One of the powerful things that helps us get to sleep is a conditioned response to our environment. It's possible that what the supplements are doing for people, on one level, is serving as a symbol of that transition. And that's where the ritual of the wind down comes in.

## Choose Your Own Wind-Down Adventure

People who come into our sleep clinic tend to have a lot of complicated problems. They've usually exhausted all of the easier routes for improving sleep. To arrive at our clinic, you'll have to have been referred by a physician and waited on the wait list, which is unfortunately several months long. So when we see people with sleep problems, they've typically been struggling for quite a long time.

Billie is a woman who came to the sleep clinic with insom-

nia. The lack of an effective wind down wasn't her only problem. As with all our patients, we engaged in the full suite of
interventions, including cognitive behavioral therapy for insomnia, setting a consistent wake-up time (which we talked
about in day one), and stimulus control and sleep restriction
(which we'll discuss in days six and seven!). But we did focus in
on creating a wind-down ritual that was really going to work
for her, because as a self-described "night owl" type, it was
something she struggled with. She tended to just *keep going*. A
complicating factor was that Billie had severe migraines. Sometimes, when she had a bad one, she'd end up having to spend the
whole day in bed. That made it extra hard for her to shift into
low gear and transition into sleep that night. We had to work
really hard to try to shift her circadian rhythm so that she could
more reliably fall asleep at night, even after a bad health day.

"The most effective wind-down activity is going to be something you enjoy, but that's also relaxing," I told her. "Anything
come to mind?"

She thought about it. "You know, I do love to cross-stitch,"
she said. "It's hard to find the time to do it, but I'd love to do it
more. And I definitely find it relaxing."

*Great*, I thought. *Cross-stitch sounds pretty boring—perfect!*

When she came in a week later, I asked her how things were
going.

"Oh, terribly!" she said rather cheerfully. "I've been staying
up all night. I think it's actually gotten worse."

I quizzed her on what was going on. At first, she simply

claimed that her "night owl" tendencies were getting the better of her. But as I questioned more, it turned out that she was pulling all-nighters because she'd gotten so involved in her cross-stitch projects.

"Sure, I'm not sleeping," she said. "But look at all these projects I've finished!"

She started flipping through pictures on her phone of canvas after canvas of elaborate scenes.

I sighed.

For me, cross-stitch would have put me to sleep immediately. For Billie, it was creative and stimulating. She got into an energizing flow. The last thing she wanted to do once she got going was go to bed. As we'd say in the sleep clinic, her "dopaminergic reward pathway" was on overdrive: the activity was just too rewarding.

Billie wasn't the only case where the wind down I've recommended turned out to be anything but. I've recommended reading, but to a bookworm, that's a reason to burn the candle at both ends. I've recommended meditation, only to have patients with anxiety tell me that it only made their intrusive nighttime thoughts even louder. So now, when I talk to people about what to do, I don't give them any specific activities at all. I tell them the feelings we're trying to accomplish, and the feelings we're trying to avoid, and have them generate the activities for themselves, with the goal of allowing the mind and body to relax, leaving the door open for sleep to come in.

After the failed wind down with Billie, I drew a simple diagram on the whiteboard for her:

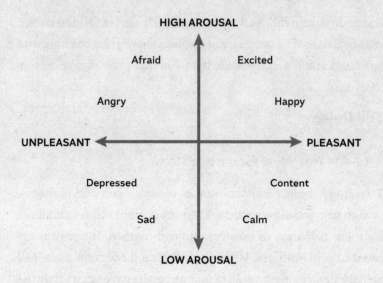

At the top of the diagram, you'll see our "high arousal" states; the bottom half represents our "low arousal" states. High energy at the top, low energy at the bottom. Meanwhile, the left and right hemispheres capture pleasant and unpleasant emotions. Slice it both ways, and you can map any of the various states we might find ourselves in physiologically throughout the day, due to various dynamic factors in our environment and inner world. "Excited" and "calm" are both positive emotions, but on opposite sides of the spectrum in arousal. "Sad" and "calm," meanwhile, are both low arousal, but on opposite sides of the emotional spectrum. Low arousal isn't great if you're weeping into your chamomile tea. The sweet spot is that lower right-hand wedge, of *positive low arousal*: Calm. Grateful. Tranquil. Content. Anything that can help get you there gets my stamp of approval. As I mentioned, it's very individual. But within that individual menu of options, there are some hard and fast rules you'll need to abide by if you want this to work.

## The Rules

### Set Aside Two Hours for the Wind Down

Two hours before bedtime (or as close as you can manage), switch to wind-down mode. I tell my patients to set an alarm for their goal time so they can make it happen. It's easy to get caught up in stuff and let the cutoff time blow right past. Tell Siri or Alexa to alert you. If you happen to have smart lighting in your home, program the lights to dim down around this time. Not only will it cue the transition, but it will also limit light exposure, allowing your melatonin system to get working. When you get the cue that it's time to wind down from whatever type of alert or alarm you choose, there are a few big-ticket items that you really do have to stop pretty immediately, which I've outlined next.

### Stop Doing Work

This one's a dealbreaker. I don't care how much you love your work—it will never serve you during your wind-down window. Any kind of work is going to keep you, at best, in the positive high-arousal sector, if not the negative high-arousal sector (I like my job, but when I'm up late grinding through emails and crunching numbers, I definitely start to veer into the negative, high-arousal wedge of our graph above). Look—if you have to pull a late night for work every so often, it's fine. Such is life. I pulled an all-nighter recently in the lab because we were running a sleep study where we had to monitor the sleeper all night long. By the time the sun came up, I was so jumpy that I leapt out of my seat when the hood of my own sweatshirt startled me.

If you're regularly working into the night, and feeling terrible and having sleep problems, then, well, work's your problem, and it's probably something you're going to have to deal with in some way to make a change. But a lot of the time, the stuff we're trying to cram in at night could more easily be accomplished the next day, when we're rested and sharper. Or, it's just not that critical that it's worth chipping away at your health over. Zoom out and ask yourself: Does this absolutely need to get done *tonight*? What are the consequences? Are there tasks that can be postponed to protect your sleep time? Getting perspective really does help.

### Stop Social Media

A lot of people will insist that they find social media relaxing. Sorry, you do not. But let's admit it, for many of us, your smartphone is the last thing you put down at night and the first thing you pick up in the morning. I get it—I succumb to this, too, but I really try to put it down at night because I know how bad it is for my sleep. The phone really becomes a problem for people—one of the most helpful things you can do in the hours leading up to bedtime is get your phone away from you. Plug it in at a charging station in another room from wherever you're going to be. Studies have shown that having your phone even nearby impacts your attention and cognitive processes.[4]

There's a little wiggle room here: if you're checking in on family, or connecting with faraway friends you really enjoy, a little social-media time can be a great way to mellow out and start feeling better about the world. But you need to be careful here. These apps were designed to capture and keep your attention—it's hard to break away, even when you realize they're having a negative effect. And even if the effect isn't negative, these apps can still work powerfully against sleep: social media has been shown to cause dopamine surges in the brain.[5] So if you're scrolling social media and doing a lot of comparing (*his life looks better than mine*) or catching up on the news (I don't know about you, but most of the breaking news these days does not bring down my arousal levels) you're going to need to cut it off. You can catch up on the news another time, you can get your daily dose of doomscrolling in the morning, those hilarious Tik-Tok videos aren't going anywhere (the internet is forever!), and as for comparison, just remember that no one's life is perfect, and what we see on Instagram is very carefully curated.

So sure: message some friends, put hearts on their posts, enjoy the pictures of their spaghetti-smeared babies. But then, disconnect. Don't let this suck up all your downtime. The bottom line: you have to disconnect.

## Stop Drinking

There's one very commonly used wind-down tactic that univer-sally goofs people up. I hate to break the news to all you night-cap enthusiasts, but it's *alcohol*.

Honestly, alcohol seems like a great wind down. It mellows you out. It's calming. Used in moderation, it does tend to put you in that low-arousal/positive-emotion wedge of the graph. Alco-hol is a soporific—it does help people relax, and can help them fall asleep, which is why roughly one in ten people end up rely-ing on it as a falling-to-sleep aid. No surprise that alcohol sales increased 20 percent during the first six months of the COVID-19 pandemic.[6] It's kind of like taking an Ambien...except it doesn't work as well. In fact, it backfires.

Alcohol is a central nervous system depressant: basically, it slows brain activity down. Alcohol is a small molecule that, once consumed, enters the bloodstream and can easily shimmy its way across the blood-brain-barrier to affect the brain. It then binds itself to your GABA receptors, which leads to feelings of relaxation and sleepiness. Sounds effective, right? Well, here's the problem: hours after the party's over, and you're snoozing away in bed, the alcohol wears off. The capacity of your GABA receptors to produce relaxation and sleep stops. You move into a lighter phase of sleep or even wake up completely, and find yourself tossing and turning in the dark.

Alcohol affects your sleep architecture by suppressing REM sleep. Typically, if you recall, you go through about somewhere between four and six sleep cycles over the course of a night, each one with a segment of REM, or rapid eye movement sleep—that's the sleep where you do your dreaming. What happens with alcohol is that it suppresses REM in the first half of the night, so you get a disproportionately long period of deep sleep early on. Then in the second half, when the alcohol starts to wear off, you get a "REM rebound" to make up for what was suppressed. The consequence of this—in tandem with the fading of GABA receptor activity—is that people get fragmented sleep. They wake up a lot in the second half of the night. The sleep they do get doesn't feel as restorative. Thankfully, this isn't permanent for the vast majority of us—however, in chronic alcoholism, it can change the brain to the point where even after you discontinue drinking, your sleep may never really be the same.

So . . . can you still drink? Sure! I'm not the fun police (though my patients have insisted otherwise at times). From a sleep perspective it can just come down to timing, and of course quantity—know that overindulging may very well have sleep consequences. Keep it light, keep it early. If you want to, go for the European vibe and have your glass of wine at lunch. If anyone looks at you askance, just tell them a sleep scientist told you to do it. Or, make sure you squeeze in your end-of-the-day wine, beer, or cocktail well before wind-down time. Alcohol is metabolized at a rate where if you have a drink several hours before bedtime (roughly three hours) it's unlikely to make much of a difference to your sleep. The problem is nightcaps, overuse, and if you're using it *to fall* asleep.

So this week: no alcohol for at least three hours before you go to bed. And if you accept, I'd like to offer you a further challenge: no alcohol at all. Try it out. See if it makes a difference in your sleep. We have an amazing capacity to run our own, personalized sleep-science experiment. You're in the middle of gathering data on yourself: why not get another data point? You may find this makes a huge difference for you . . . or that it doesn't make much of a dent. Either way, it's worth finding out.

## Recipe for a Great Wind Down

The point in stopping all of the above is that you unplug from the day, to give yourself the opportunity to let cognitive arousal dissipate. It's not really something you can rush—you have to allow it to happen.

Again, this is an individual process, and you'll pick what works for you. But there are a few heavy-hitter wind-down activities that tend to work for people across the board. In brief:

- *Take a bath or a shower.* It's not your imagination that these help with sleep. A warm bath or hot shower helps because it facilitates your core body temperature cooling, which is one of the things that happens as you get sleepy. Hot water aids in natural thermoregulation: your body warms up, and then when you get out, the water evaporates from your skin, cooling your body more quickly and signaling your brain that it's time to sleep. It can also be a powerful signal: a ritual that cues your body that bedtime is coming. It's relaxing, it leaves people with a clean feeling that helps them relax and let go, it clearly marks a transition from "being alert" to "resting."

- **Read or watch TV.** I always give people this option, as much as books and websites will say not to. I see people all the time who've gotten advice where TV was off the table, and they say, "It was so tortuous and anxiety-provoking, sitting in my living room with my thoughts, trying to relax!" Books are great, but not everyone's a reader. One caveat: this isn't an excuse to start binge-watching the next thrilling series you've been so excited to watch. *Excited* is not what we're going for, remember? Shows you've already seen, or that are more on the mellow end and won't keep you hooked in episode after episode—that's what we're going for. Important note: if you choose reading or watching TV as your wind-down activity, *do not do this in bed*. (We'll discuss why in the next chapter.)

- **Deep breathing.** Breathing can engage the parasympathetic nervous system—also called the "rest and digest" system. To fall asleep, we need to disengage the fight-or-flight response. Anything that dampens down the sympathetic nervous system (stress response) and powers up the parasympathetic (relaxation, connection) is going to work here. And certain types of breathing have been proven to "activate" the parasympathetic arm of the nervous system. One popular exercise is called Resonance Frequency Breathing. Heart rate and respiration tend to be in sync, or in resonance, at around 6 breaths per minute (actually 5.5 breaths/minute). The goal here is to take slow belly breaths, inhaling through your nose for about five seconds, and then slowly exhale, either through your nose or pursed lips, for another five seconds.

Those are just a few of my top picks. You have two hours—do all three! Or pick from the menu I offer my patients:

- Dim the lights
- Nightly meditation
- A gratitude journal
- Watch a show or a movie
- Read
- Take bath or shower
- Sit outside and look at the stars
- Listen to a podcast
- Anything that makes you feel positive

## Customize Your Own List

Take a moment now to brainstorm the kinds of activities that would work for *you* during a wind down tonight. It's also sometimes instructive to identify which activities might *not* work. The typical stuff that shows up on a list of ways to relax before bed might not work for you. (Remember Billie and her cross-stitch!) Use the chart below to map the activities you generally do in the evening, and be realistic about where they'd accurately appear. For instance, "work" would probably be in the high-arousal upper half, but depending on your job and mood, it could go in either the unpleasant side or the pleasant quadrant! "Taking a relaxing bath" would probably go in low-arousal/pleasant. What goes in the low-arousal/positive quadrant, for you personally? Write down as many ideas as you can think of.

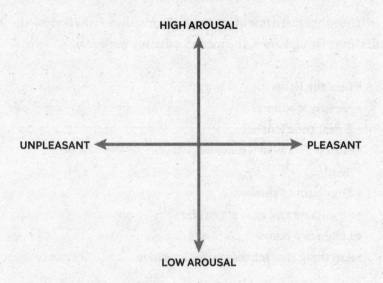

## You Can't Have It All . . . but You Can Have the Most Important Thing

The wind down isn't about specifically what you do. It's that you have to make the time. The bottom line is: You can't have it all. You will not be able to go full tilt right until you want to turn off, and then get great sleep. It's either/or.

With Omar, the computer programmer from the beginning of this chapter, we did finally get to a schedule that worked for him. He said that he didn't have the time for a wind down. I said, "Make the time, or you will not achieve your goal of going off your sleep meds and sleeping well."

He simply had to choose what was more important to him.

He chose sleep.

We agreed that he would stop working earlier in the evening, watch Netflix (*not* in his bed—more on this tomorrow), and then take his meds at 11 p.m. He was able to reliably fall asleep "on time" by about midnight, and could wake up to drive his wife to work without stressing about lost sleep. Then we tapered down the meds. When we wean people off medications like Ambien, we do an every-other-day progression: you take your usual 10 mg, then the next day, take 5 mg; then back to 10 mg, then back to 5 mg. If this works, then we bump down to shifting between 5 mg and 2.5 mg . . . and so on. We only progress when people report that they're still doing well. We rarely have to move backward. This tapering typically happens while the patient incorporates all of the techniques described in this book, especially the ones I'll describe in the next chapters. When all of these tools are used together, we find that for most patients, they don't even notice the dosage dropping. They're reclaiming their natural ability to fall asleep.

For the vast majority of people with insomnia struggles, the biggest challenge is behavioral. It's our habit to work late. It's our routine to scroll on the phone. We have entrenched beliefs that we should be busy and productive. When that wind-down alarm goes off, our instinct is to rationalize and say, "Tonight I need to keep working (or doing x); it's too important." So when your phone buzzes you that it's wind-down time tonight, and every night this week, I want you to remind yourself that this wind-down time is in service of better sleep. And with better sleep, you have better learning, creativity, attention, and memory. You can task-switch more smoothly and efficiently. You're better at emotional regulation. People who get good sleep have better relationships with their spouses. Sleep regulates your metabolism—people who have short sleep over a long period of time gain more weight, and crave less nutritious food.[7] There have been fascinating studies on sleep and leadership, and how it affects how well you treat your employees and how empathetic and collaborative you are.[8]

Think about the long game. Maintaining a solid level of sleep health will serve you so much better in the long term than whatever your immediate pressing issue is right now. It's a much better investment in your health and well-being to protect your sleep as opposed to always putting out fires in your life and treating *life* and *sleep* like they're two separate things. A lot of living happens while you're sleeping—all kinds of restoration and preparation for the daylight hours. We have this unfortunate compartmentalization around sleep and life, but they're interconnected, all part of the same experience.

And: continue prioritizing this wind down even if it doesn't lead to the most amazing night of sleep every time. You will probably still have nights where you struggle. None of us are ever guaranteed perfect sleep, no matter how perfectly we set ourselves up. But if you maintain these practices, your sleep *is* going to gradually improve. If you stick with it, even when you have a bad night, your sleep will be better and your life will be better.

## TODAY'S PRACTICE

# SLOW DOWN TO SHUT DOWN

### Know the Ground Rules

Remember the first important instruction: start your wind down at *least* two hours before bed! No exceptions this week. If you're working on your sleep and want to see improvement, this is essential. And second: don't do your wind down in bed. We'll talk more about why in the next chapter, but for now, just know that it could undermine your sleep later on if you spend too much time in bed leading up to bedtime.

### Set an Alarm

You need an alarm for your wind down just like you need one to wake up. When it goes off, *no snoozing!* Wrap up whatever you're doing. If it helps open again to this page and remind yourself why you need to . . .

### Prioritize It

This is how you can be creative, productive, smart, and *emotionally* smart. Not now, when you're cognitively depleted, but tomorrow. Save the late nights and all-nighters of work for rare occasions when it's really and truly critical. (If this is a regular necessity for you, let me tell you as a clinician who's seen in the impact of short sleep on people's health, right down to their immune cells, that it's time to make a change.) Sleep is money in the bank, and also for your brain, your body, your health and longevity, your relationships, and your capacity to enjoy your life. So transition out of work mode and . . .

### Pick Your Potion!

As we learned in this chapter, not every recommended wind down is a wind down for *you*. Choose from the options we went through, or pull an idea from the chart you filled out—just remember that we're shooting for activities that put you in that sweet-spot quadrant of pleasant, calm, low arousal. You have two hours to fill. What are you choosing? Go forth and unwind!

### Troubleshooting

#### If you're still wound up at the end of your wind down . . .

A couple things to think about if this is the case. Number one, pay attention to your body. I have had people who are oblivious to their sleepiness cues. It's been so long since they've allowed themselves to pay attention to them that they've lost track of what they look and feel like. Along with that, there's this idea people have that there's a particular "window of time" that they need to be in bed by. They go by that, rather than really tapping into their body.

I had one patient who would actually notice that she was feeling sleepy but would "push through" to do the full two-hour wind down. Don't do this! Part of winding down is paying attention to your senses (another great reason not to do anything too engaging, like a new television show or social media—you get sucked in and can't pay attention to your body anymore).

Finally, if the wind down isn't working magic for you, don't give up on it. It will take some *repetition* of this ritual for your body to learn to regard the wind down as a cue for sleep. Tomorrow's practice is going to tackle this head-on.

# DAY 6

## (RE)TRAIN YOUR BRAIN

**TODAY IS THE DAY YOU BEGIN TO TRAIN YOURSELF, LIKE A PET DOG.** In fact, like Pavlov's dog.

In the 1890s, Ivan Pavlov, a Russian physiologist, was studying conditional reflexes in animals: the instinctual physical responses we have to certain stimuli. When food is presented to an animal, it will salivate in response. Pavlov wanted to study the secretion of various fluids throughout the gastrointestinal system in response to eating, so he inserted a small saliva collection tube in the dog's cheek. When food was given to the dog, an assistant would monitor and measure the saliva. But then he noticed something. The dogs didn't salivate in response to the food being put down in front of them, as you'd expect from a conditional reflex. They salivated at the sound of the assistant's feet as he brought the food. They had learned to strongly associate footsteps in the hallway with being fed—so much so that their mouths watered in anticipation at the sound of shoes outside the door, whether or not any food was forthcoming.

He ran more experiments, quickly training the dogs to salivate in response to a clicking metronome, and then to a bell. He found that as long as he presented the two stimuli to the dogs (the food, the sound) close enough together in time, the dogs would quickly build an association between the two things. He called this the "conditioned response": the previously neutral stimulus (bell) meant nothing to the dogs, but after conditioning, they had a new, instinctual response to the sound.[1]

The key to "classical conditioning" and the conditioned response is that it hooks a trigger to an already existing physiological response. The body has all kinds of conditioned responses to various triggers throughout the day. We've already talked about some: for example, with a stable and consistent wake time, your body will produce cortisol *in anticipation of* your wake-up time. Some others: when you drink a glass of water, your thirst is quenched immediately, long before the water has been processed through your system and added to your bodily fluids. When you take a sip of coffee, you may feel immediately perkier, even though that caffeine still has a long road before the chemicals affect your brain. This is happening all the time . . . whether you're aware of it or not.

## You Are Pavlov's Dog

We often don't appreciate the importance of our environment and routine. Our surroundings have become second nature, and day-to-day routines are often shaped by forces outside our control that we adapt to: work schedules, school schedules, commutes, the rhythms and demands of the communities where we live. Through all of this, the brain is constantly taking in information, keeping track of what's coming up, anticipating demands, and telling the body how it should use its metabolic resources. Your brain wants your body to be efficient. It wants to optimize. So it develops heuristics, or shortcuts based on repeated behaviors.

Before the pandemic disrupted routines almost everywhere, I used to arrive home from the lab at the same time every evening—right when it was time to eat dinner. Then suddenly, everything changed. We couldn't have everyone in the lab together, so our schedules had to adapt. I was arriving home late at night, or in the middle of the afternoon. But as soon as my hand touched the doorknob of our apartment, I felt immediately hungry. It didn't matter what time I got home—my body had a conditioned response to my apartment door. Turning that doorknob meant it was time to eat. No matter that it was actually 2 a.m. after a long shift, and that I'd already eaten—my body's conditioned response was, "Quick! Start making insulin!"

The same is true for your bed. Your bed can be an incredibly powerful stimulus for sleep—*if* your body is conditioned to respond to it as such. For people who don't have any sleep problems, the process is smooth: before they go to bed, their circadian rhythm is right where it needs to be. Their sleep pressure is high. And the act of getting into bed itself is like this hammer that drops, this final amount of weight and pressure that allows them to drop right into sleep. Unfortunately, for those with sleep struggles, it frequently turns out that they've built the *opposite* conditioned response to their bed.

## The Dark Side of the Conditioned Response

"You know, Dr. Prather, I was feeling really sleepy, and then I got in bed and my brain woke up!"

I hear this all the time in the sleep clinic. When people have chronic sleep issues, it frequently turns out to be the case that they've established a conditioned response to the bed that's the exact opposite of what we want. They describe feeling like "a switch had flipped" as soon as they climbed in bed—suddenly, they were alert. This is called *conditioned arousal*: the bed itself has become a trigger for an active, restless mind. And it's 100 percent because your body is now confused. It's spent so much time in bed awake, dreading sleep, trying to sleep, having difficult, anxious thoughts, that it's begun to associate the bed with this wakefulness and angst. And that conditioning is extremely powerful—as powerful as the bell that made the dog's mouth water on command.

Your conditioned response is now working *against* sleep. So the first thing we need to do is break apart that conditioning. We need to kill the association between anxious wakefulness and the bed.

## Breaking Down Conditioned Arousal

Pavlov's dogs associated the sound of that bell so strongly to the arrival of food, their bodies would launch into the digestive process as soon as they heard it ring. But breaking that conditioned response, Pavlov found, was just as easy, if you were consistent. Ring that bell over and over again and offer no food, and pretty quickly, the conditioned response would fade away. The dogs heard the bell but had no reaction. The brain and body learned, and adapted—the stimulus and the response were unhooked from each other once again.

We began this week with the number-one instruction that I give people who want to improve their sleep: stabilize your wake time and stick to it. This is number 2: *don't get in bed unless you're sleepy and if you can't sleep, get up.* These two strategies together are, in my experience as a sleep scientist, the double-whammy, two most powerful changes we can make to help ourselves sleep better. When you remove yourself from the bed when you can't sleep, you begin to break the association your body has between *in bed* and *on alert.* Your body has learned this response; it can unlearn it.

This conditioned response, that *bed* equals *awake and anxious,* is at the foundation of most insomnia. Partly, it's because the solution feels so counterintuitive. The idea of the conditioned response makes sense to people when I explain it, sure. But when it actually comes time to *get up out of bed,* late at night in the dark, that's another story.

Even the patients I have with the worst insomnia, who

desperately want better sleep, will have resistance to this tactic—even though it's one of the most powerful tools in the good-sleep toolbox. So I want to take you through a few of the major points of concern about this method.

*People say:* "It sucks to get up at night!"

Yeah, it's definitely unpleasant to have to get out of your nice, warm, comfy bed. But there's truly nothing else that can replace this act in terms of teaching your body to sleep.

*People say:* "It wakes me up more if I get up and move around."

Trust me, it doesn't. You are already awake. All you're doing by staying in bed is reinforcing the association between lying in bed and being awake. You're teaching your body to respond to your bed with alertness and wakefulness. It does feel counterintuitive—it can feel like getting up is giving up. But when you're going through a period of deconditioning your learned arousal, it's the exact right thing to do.

*People say:* "I'll be able to fall asleep if I can just think through this problem."

When we can't fall asleep, or wake up in the middle of the night, we're susceptible to anxious thoughts and ruminative looping. Certainly we can try some of the tactics we discussed earlier, like "trainspotting" and distraction, but if these thought patterns are happening alongside conditioned arousal, that's going to be an uphill battle—and maybe not a winnable one. It becomes a reason that people stay in bed far longer than they should: they end up trying to "figure out the thinking" of why they're having anxious thoughts, or what they can do about their worries. It makes sense as an impulse (we are incessant problem solvers) but it's hard to address these kinds of things in the middle of the night when we're already taxed. That's why we try to move that kind of thinking out of nighttime and into scheduled time during the next day, as we talked about in the previous chapter.

**People say:** "If I get up now, it will just make things worse tomorrow."

This is probably the toughest one to overcome. It's easy to start catastrophizing about the sleep we're losing as we work on this. In the middle of the night, when you're at your most vulnerable, everything seems dire—especially if you're operating on a sleep deficit. Watching the clock squeeze our potential sleep time into a smaller and smaller wedge of time, we get overwhelmed with extreme thoughts about how we'll feel tomorrow if we don't fall asleep *now*.

I'm going to feel terrible.

I won't be able to keep my eyes open all day.

I'm going to bomb the job interview if I don't fall asleep in the next five minutes.

It's ironic: so often, the thing that really gets in our way when it comes to sleep is this feeling of *urgency* to fall asleep, borne of all these consequences we imagine happening the next day. Yes—losing sleep has consequences, as we've discussed. But the ramifications of a couple bad nights are almost never as bad as we imagine. These types of thoughts are fantastic at prolonging our inability to fall asleep, and they just aren't accurate.

One of my current patients, Jasmine, is a very driven young woman. Until recently, she held a high-powered corporate position. She worked long and demanding hours, but she loved excelling in that world. Then, she had a stroke.

She's recovered, but it's been a process. The stroke knocked her out of the workforce, and off the track she was on. She lost ground in her career, which for her, is a huge concern and point of stress. She's still rehabilitating, and part of it is relearning to sleep. Some of the treatments she underwent involved medications that can disrupt circadian rhythms and cause sleep issues. Something like that can start someone down the path of conditioned arousal as they spend too much time in bed trying and failing to fall asleep. And for Jasmine, who feels like so much is riding on every Zoom meeting and phone call, it can be really hard to stave off those anxious thoughts that make sleep even more elusive. So, we've spent a lot of time doing "thought records"—she writes down the stuff she's thinking in the middle of the night, and then we look at the evidence about how she felt and performed the next day. It makes it a little easier to see that these thoughts aren't usually correct. Our thoughts shape our emotions, and so if we're being tyrannized by untrue beliefs in the middle of the night, it's time to bust these myths we're telling ourselves.

It's a lot harder for thoughts like these to dominate our nights when we can look at the data and say, "Hey, actually, it wasn't that bad!" When we go over thought records with patients in the sleep clinic, we get as granular as possible: What's true and what's not true about this thought? Is this thought helpful? What's the evidence for *and against* these ideas?

Jasmine found that while she maybe wasn't her sharpest after a bad night of sleep, none of the horrible things she imagined ever came to pass. Nobody noticed or remarked upon poor job performance. She got everything essential done. She also found that sometimes when she *did* get a great night of sleep, it wasn't her most amazing day at work, either. So maybe her job performance wasn't as tightly tied to her sleep as she believed it was. Just being able to loosen the grip of that sleep anxiety a little bit helped her get out of her own way at night.

She's working in consulting currently, trying to get back into her field slowly. A lot of the consulting she's doing, though, is pretty high stakes, involving big mergers. Recently, she was going into an important call the next day, and just could not sleep the night before. When she reported back to me later, her assessment was that she didn't sleep "at all." She had to just push through the call on zero sleep, but she did it. "Look at that," I said. "The worst thing happened, and you made it through."

We built on this, and worked on coming up with phrases she could use to remind herself that this had worked out in the past. "It'll be fine, it wasn't that bad last time." "I've gotten through this before." What you want is a shortcut to the feeling of calm; to the deep knowledge that you will be OK, even if you lose some sleep time. You don't want to be thinking through it and problem solving in the middle of the night—you work on it during the day, so that you can *recall* it in the middle of the night.

So, the next time you're in bed and stressed about being unable to fall asleep, remember that it will be OK. But the key here is that when you're awake and mentally aroused, you need to physically get out of bed. What I advise people to do is to go back to one of their wind-down activities. Then, when you feel sleepy again, return to bed. If you immediately wake up again? You guessed it. Up again. What you're here doing is "re-pairing" the feeling of sleepiness with the bed itself. You're putting the food bowl down on the ground and ringing the bell, over and over again, until your body begins to respond.

The bottom line: There isn't a better way. You can't think yourself to sleep. The only way to replace conditioned arousal with a different response is to *do* it, repeatedly and consistently, until your body has adapted. And *it will*.

## Stimulus Control: the Key Piece of the Sleep Puzzle

Everything we've been working on this week is part of what we call CBTI, or *cognitive behavioral therapy for insomnia*. Cognitive behavioral therapy is a psychological and behavioral treatment that's used to treat a whole range of things, from depression, to anxiety, to sleep. The central tenet here is that thoughts, behaviors, and emotions are all linked. Often, the sleep problems we encounter stem from learned patterns of unhelpful behaviors. What I mean by "unhelpful behaviors" is that you've learned ways of coping (with life, with stress, with all kinds of challenges) that don't serve you very well. Perhaps they make intuitive sense in the moment, but they undermine your health and well-being in the long term.

As we saw above with Jasmine, a lot of people struggle because they've developed this disordered thinking around sleep. Anxiety about sleep becomes the very thing that sabotages our ability to sleep. But what's fascinating about insomnia is that, more so than other issues like, say, depression, it has a strong behavioral component to it. To be clear: I do not mean that people are to blame for their insomnia—so many of our habits and behaviors are borne of necessity, to cope with schedules, stress, parenting, jobs, our environment, and more. The fact that insomnia is behavior-borne is a *hopeful* thing. It means that if we give people the knowledge and the tools and a clear path forward, they can indeed change their sleep. So as a clinician, my approach has always been to first deal with all of the accessible behavior things, and *then* tackle the disordered beliefs around sleep. This stuff can be tough to break through. But if we can get you sleeping a little bit better through these simple, straightforward behavior adjustments, then you will very likely begin to develop a sense of "sleep mastery" on your own. And some of that sleep anxiety just begins to naturally fall away.

That's why we're focusing on these behavioral basics that you can do immediately and that have a big impact: like *stimulus control*, which is what we've been talking about and what you're going to start doing today. Because one of our major behavior-based problems is that we have this broken relationship with our bed. We've eroded that strong association we once had of *bed* with *sleep*. So when we fix this, we can cut down so much of the other stuff—like anxious thought patterns—that keep us awake at night.

I don't want you to feel bad when you hear that most sleep problems are behavior-based. I want you to feel empowered. The more you know—the more you understand about what works and why, and how and why your body responds to your environment and routine—the more you'll be able to intervene, and the easier everything will feel.

When I see people in the clinic, I get them started on stimulus control right away. There's a lot we can't do yet for people when they first come in—we need to send them home with their sleep diary (like the one you've been keeping), have them collect their data, and then come back in and evaluate. At that point, we figure out the best interventions. The thing about stimulus control is that it works universally. It's important, it's powerful, and you can start immediately. So with patients, I don't wait. I'm not sure yet what will be the specific path forward for each individual, but I do know that it will involve today's practice.

### TODAY'S PRACTICE

# MAKE YOUR BED THE SLEEP TRIGGER

If you have a conditioned-arousal problem, you're in good company. The vast majority of people we see in the sleep clinic struggle with this and need to practice what we call "stimulus control." I said today you were going to train your brain like Pavlov's dog, so here's how you do it.

### Rule #1: Do Not Get into Your Bed Until You're Sleepy

Remember, you're starting your wind down roughly two hours before bedtime. But be aware of your own body. You don't need to be rigid about this. If two hours is up and you're still wide awake, keep on winding down! Remember, as much as we'd love to have more control, we don't get to decide when we fall asleep. Sleep comes to you. So, downshift into something even less stimulating. For example, if you've been reading, maybe relax with your eyes closed and listen to music. (I recommend meditating here, if that's your thing.)

### Rule #2: Don't Do Other Things in Your Bed

No phone, no laptop, no book. Bed is for sleep and sex only. (Caveat: it won't always be this way. You aren't doomed to never-Netflix in your comfy bed for the rest of your days. But when you're trying to fix this, be as clear to your body as you possibly can. No mixed messages.)

### Rule #3: Give It a Shot

You get in bed, you feel sleepy, but you're not falling asleep yet. That's OK. Give it a chance! Let's say, fifteen minutes. It often takes people between fifteen and twenty minutes to fall asleep—this is completely normal. I want you to give yourself an honest chance here: this is not a "watching the clock like a hawk" fifteen minutes. Try the visualization exercise from page 86: fill up that working memory with something pleasant and vivid. If random thoughts are keeping you from letting go, try "trainspotting."

### Rule #4: If You're Up, Get Up!

If you've followed rule #3 above and hit the twenty- to thirty-minute mark of lying in bed, it is time to get out of bed. Get up and transition back to wind-down mode. Go read your book. Listen to smooth jazz. Smell some candles. Drink some tea. When you feel that sweet sleepy feeling again, get back in bed.

Notice: I'm not telling you to go sit alone in a dark room! You have tools at your disposal to wind down. But there are some important don'ts. Don't flip on all the lights—we want you to keep that melatonin humming along. Don't use this time to be more efficient with your life—this is not a moment to knock out emails or blast through those left-over dishes. This is part of your practice toward improving your sleep. When you have to get up at night as part of your sleep conditioning, that "up" time becomes part of your wind down. Protect it.

### Rule #5: Stick with It!

Do this practice not just tonight, but tomorrow, and the next night. This isn't going to work overnight. It works over time. Pavolv's dogs physically associated the sound of footsteps with the arrival of food because they internalized a pattern. We need your body to internalize this pattern, which means you need to make it a pattern! Consistency and repetition are key. It can take a couple of weeks for this to start working. Results can vary—you aren't a robot, everybody's different. Even Pavlov and his assistants found big variations between the dogs' responses. Their individual personalities and proclivities affected their response to conditioning. There's no particular deadline or benchmark for success here. But if you're doing this consistently, *along with* the other strategies we've been practicing (this is important: in the lab, all of these tactics are practiced in concert with each other, not individually) you'll see results.

And if you wake up in the middle of the night (we all do, way more times than we think we do, we just often don't remember it) then the same rules above apply. Don't stay in bed past twenty minutes or so, just because it's 3 a.m. Remember what you want your body to learn: that *bed* equals *sleepiness*. We know from sleep studies that this will work: if you practice stimulus control consistently, the bed will become a *helpful* sleep trigger for you instead of a location of struggle or anxiety. Soon, lying in your bed will cause physiological changes in your body that will allow sleep to occur more easily. The bed itself can become your portal to sleep.

## Troubleshooting

### What If I Can't Get out of Bed?

This is a frequent and valid issue. I work with people who are at risk of falling at night. People who have chronic pain and can't move around much. People who live in studio apartments, where their bed is the only place to sit in the entire apartment, and they really have no place else to be *but* the bed. People who have partners who will be disturbed by all this up and down.

In these cases, we go to the underlying principle: make the experience *different* from lying in bed and trying to fall asleep. Do everything you can to give your body clear cues that *this is not sleeping*.

If you can't get out of bed, here are some alternative strategies I frequently recommend:

- Sit all the way up! Make it clear from your posture and positioning that you are no longer in "sleep mode."
- Move to the other side of the bed! You can wind down a foot away and then "go back to bed" on your regular side. (When I was a kid, I used to flip upside down to read in bed, then flip back up to go to sleep. I guess I've always been a sleep scientist. . . .)

### When You Have a Partner . . .

It can be challenging when you're worried about waking someone up. I don't like to use the phrase "sleep divorce"— it sounds way too dire and final! But consider going on a "sleep break" if you're lying in bed awake because you're reluctant to disturb your sleeping partner. That's just more of a recipe for continued arousal. Do your reconditioning in the guest room if you have one . . . or if your partner is an easier sleeper, maybe they can sleep in the guest room as a gift to you!

The other issue has to do with values and how people spend their free time, which can be closely tied to identity and expressions of love. I've had a number of couples who like to get in bed together and read or watch a show at night—it's a special time for them, and a part of their daily routine that they treasure. The idea that we use the bed only for sleeping is inconsistent with these other values they have.

I had one couple like this—I'll call them Ellie and Spencer. They were in their late sixties, both retired, but busy. They spent their days helping out with their grandchildren and volunteering with community organizations. For years it had been their habit to get in bed together early in the evening and read the current periodicals, trading articles back and forth. They didn't want to give it up.

"Can't we do everything else, but keep this? It's like doing a wind down anyway," they said.

"Of course, it's your choice," I said. "That's totally fine and sounds lovely. But look, the reality is, you can't have everything. You're here because you're struggling with sleep. So it may be the case that you can't have this particular part of your routine, and good sleep. This is like a recipe: we can do all the other things, but if we don't put in the eggs, it won't come out."

You have control here, but you do have to make a choice. Is the routine you love that might be disrupted more important than improving your sleep, or less? The answer will be personal. And framing it as a choice instead of something that's just happening to you helps us see that we can make trade-offs depending on what we value. Maybe it does take you longer to fall asleep for this reason or that reason, but if you can come to a degree of acceptance and not have distress over it, it's OK. It works for you: "This is a choice I'm making because I value this time with my partner." But maybe it's worth pursuing a creative solution. Ellie and Spencer liked to relax in bed together because the rest of the house made them feel like they were "on duty"—dishes to wash, plants to water, floors to sweep, emails to reply to. The reason they loved to spend this time hanging out in the bed was that it felt like a boat on the ocean, where they were really secluded and sealed off from anything that might place demands on their attention or interrupt. What they ended up doing was setting up a comfy space in their living room that was the "evening nook," with a comfortable couch, soft blankets, and a stand-up folding screen that blocked off the rest of the house from their sight line. They were able to have exactly the same quality time together, while also preserving the "bed is for sleep" philosophy that did turn out to help them both a lot with their insomnia.

# DAY 7

## STAY UP LATE

If it was a little frustrating, I'm not surprised. Building a healthy conditioned response with your bed is much harder in the beginning. At first, it's like a dance . . . but it's not a pretty one. You feel sleepy, you get in bed, you feel awake, you get up and wait to be sleepy again, you get in bed, you feel awake. If you're feeling a little bit more tired this morning than usual after all that up and down, *good*. You can use this.

If you spent less time in bed last night, then you've rolled some sleep pressure over into today. By tonight, your sleep pressure will be naturally higher than it was last night at the exact same time. Part of why stimulus control works is that you're teaching your body to associate sleepiness with bed, as we discussed yesterday. But the other key reason it works is that you're revving up your homeostatic sleep drive. When you're lying down in bed, even if you're not asleep, there's a little relief to your sleep pressure—just resting like that does let a little air squeak out of that balloon. And this can work against you—when you experience that relief, you lose some of that pressure that helps you let go into sleep. When we ask people to get up out of bed—even when they move to a wind-down activity—it fires up the homeostatic sleep drive again. Sleep pressure builds, the balloon fills even more. Every time you go to lie back down to pair that sleepiness feeling with your bed, you have a better shot of success. And this should improve over subsequent days.

But there's an even more powerful approach to revving up the homeostatic sleep drive. It's our most effective weapon against sleep struggles that we have in the entire arsenal. It can help stabilize circadian rhythm. It can help re-pair bed with sleepiness. It can help you figure out what your ideal bedtime is, as well as your ideal total sleep time. It can allow you to feel less anxiety about sleep and more mastery over it. It can even replace sleep medication. It's called *sleep restriction*, and it boils down to this: Stay up late. Really late.

## How "Efficient" Is Your Sleep?

There's a reason we didn't begin the week with this strategy, effective though it is. We needed data first.

At the beginning of this week, I asked you to become a sleep scientist for these seven days, to conduct your own personal experiment—an at-home clinical trial where *you* are both subject and researcher. A key part of that was keeping your sleep diary, which you started on day one. By today you should have six nights of data. This is just enough for us to roughly calculate your *sleep efficiency*.

Sleep efficiency is simple: it's how much time you spend *actually* asleep compared to how much time you give yourself to sleep, i.e., your sleep opportunity.

First, let's define *sleep opportunity*. Sleep opportunity is the period of time from when you first get into bed at night to when you wake up for the last time in the morning. So even if you're practicing stimulus control as we discussed in day six and physically getting out of bed in the middle of the night if you're not sleepy, that time spent out of bed still counts as part of your sleep opportunity. Think of your sleep opportunity as a stopwatch that starts from the moment you get into bed for the first time at night, and that stops only when you wake up for the final time in the morning. It doesn't matter what happens in between—that entire period of time counts as sleep opportunity.

Now that we've understood sleep opportunity, we can discuss sleep efficiency. Sleep efficiency is measured as a percentage. Here's an example: Ben gets in bed at 10 p.m., falls asleep by 10:30 p.m., sleeps through the whole night without awakenings, and wakes to his alarm at 6 a.m. His total sleep opportunity is eight hours (480 minutes), he's asleep for seven and a half (450 minutes), and his sleep efficiency is 94 percent. Here's what that looks like as an equation, using minutes instead of hours (which is how we calculate this in the lab):

450 minutes asleep **divided by** 480 minutes of sleep opportunity = 0.9375 (94%)

That's Ben on an ideal night. Sometimes, he used to wake up in the middle of the night, around 2 a.m., and lie awake in bed for about an hour. On those nights, his sleep efficiency looked like this:

390 minutes asleep **divided by** 480 minutes of sleep opportunity = 0.8125 (82%)

Generally, what we want to see is a sleep efficiency of *at least* 85 percent, or higher. That's the threshold that we shoot for—except for with older folks, who do generally experience more fragmented sleep naturally. With people aged sixty-five and up, we shoot for a sleep efficiency of about 80 percent.

Ben's sleep efficiency is pretty good. On average, he's definitely hitting the 85 percent mark on most nights. Plus, he feels good, and doesn't struggle too much.

Ben's husband Gordon, on the other hand, has a different situation. He goes to bed with Ben at 10 p.m., but often can't fall asleep until 1 a.m. or even 2 a.m. After Ben easily drops off, Gordon reads on his phone, or switches to a book or magazine to try to keep down that blue-light exposure. He closes his eyes for a while, and when it doesn't work, he swipes his phone open again, pops in his earbuds, and watches a show or scrolls Instagram and TikTok.

When we tallied up the numbers in his sleep diary, we found the average for his time spent asleep and the average for his sleep opportunity by adding up both of those columns and dividing them by six days. His average sleep time was 305 minutes. His average sleep opportunity, like Ben's, was 480. His sleep efficiency: 64 percent. That's pretty bad.

There were a couple of things going on with Gordon. One, he wasn't practicing stimulus control the way we'd like to see— he was spending a lot of time in bed doing non-sleep and non-sex things, like watching TV, checking email on his phone, immersing himself in social media, etc. He was the first to admit that he tried all those things as ways to chill out and relax—he said that checking email to make sure there was nothing urgent there reassured him, and that scrolling Instagram relaxed him. But it was clear that he had a conditioned arousal problem—he did eventually get up, but inconsistently. He was also going to bed at the same time as Ben because it was their routine as a couple, not because he was actually sleepy at 10 p.m. That would leave him groggy the next morning, when Ben's alarm would go off and he'd wake up. Some days he got up with Ben to make coffee and chat in the kitchen before Ben headed off to work, but other days he'd go back to sleep—he was going to school to get his master's degree, and his classes didn't start until later. His wake time was also erratic. He admitted he was more of a night owl, but that his frequent sleep time of 2 a.m. was much too late. He also felt a lot of frustration and anxiety around sleep, felt he was tired and not his best at school, and that his health wasn't the greatest—he was feeling really run down. When he filled out a self-report about his health over the past few months, he did report a higher rate of colds and viruses than is typical for a healthy man his age.

We'll return to Gordon in a moment. But right now, let's take a look at *your* sleep efficiency. I'm going to teach you how to calculate your average sleep efficiency using the example below:

Please complete this to the best of your ability:

| Day of the week: | Sunday | Monday | Tuesday | Wednesday | Thursday | Friday | Saturday |
|---|---|---|---|---|---|---|---|
| Time you tried to fall asleep? | 11:45PM | 10:30PM | 12:05AM | 11:15PM | 12:30AM | 1:00AM | 12:00AM |
| How long it took you to fall asleep (in minutes)? | 15 | 45 | 20 | 25 | 10 | 5 | 30 |
| Number of times you woke up and tried to return to sleep? | 1 | 3 | 3 | 1 | 2 | 2 | 1 |
| How long were you awake during wake times reported above? (Total number of minutes) | 120 | 60 | 60 | 120 | 10 | 90 | 20 |
| Time you woke up for the last time this morning? | 6:00AM | 7:00AM | 7:00AM | 7:30AM | 6:15AM | 8:00AM | 9:00AM |
| What was your sleep quality? (0 to 100, 100 being perfect) | 70 | 40 | 50 | 30 | 75 | 40 | 70 |
| Sleep Opportunity (in minutes) | 375 | 510 | 415 | 495 | 345 | 420 | 540 |
| Time Asleep (in minutes) | 240 | 405 | 335 | 350 | 325 | 325 | 490 |
| Sleep Efficiency | 64.0% | 79.4% | 80.7% | 70.7% | 94.2% | 77.4% | 90.7% |

As you can see, sleep opportunity is the total amount of time from when you first attempt to sleep until you wake up for the last time in the morning. (Note: it could be that you are in bed for a long time prior to trying to sleep. As discussed above, you should not be getting in bed *until* you are sleepy and attempt to go to sleep.)

Time asleep is calculated by taking the sleep opportunity value and subtracting out the amount of time when you are not asleep, including the number of minutes it takes to first fall asleep and the number of minutes spent awake in the middle of the night.

Let's take a look at the example above. On Sunday, this person got into bed to go to sleep at 11:45 p.m. Though they woke up once in the middle of the night, the last time they woke up was at 6 a.m. That entire window from when they first got into bed at 11:45 p.m. until they last woke up at 6 a.m. is their sleep opportunity. The total number of minutes between 11:45 p.m. and 6 a.m. is 375 minutes. And so this person's sleep opportunity on Sunday was 375 minutes.

However, of those 375 minutes of sleep opportunity, they spent 15 minutes *trying* to fall asleep, and that awakening lasted 120 minutes in the middle of the night. So, in order to calculate time spent asleep, we take those 375 minutes of sleep opportunity they started with and subtract the 15 and 120 they spent not sleeping. This leaves us with a time asleep value of 240 minutes.

To calculate sleep efficiency, we take time asleep (240) and divide it by sleep opportunity (375), which leaves us with 0.64—a 64 percent sleep efficiency.

Knowing all this, flip back to the sleep diary pages you filled out, and tally up your sleep opportunity, your time asleep, and your sleep efficiency for each night.

Once you've calculated your sleep efficiency for every night of this past week, you can figure out your average sleep efficiency over the course of the week. If I were doing that for the example above, I'd add up all seven values in the sleep efficiency row and divide the total by seven. So, 64.0 + 79.4 + 80.7 + 70.7 + 94.2 + 77.4 + 90.7, which comes out to 557.1. Then 557.1 divided by 7 comes out to 79.6. So, the average sleep efficiency for the example above is 79.6 percent.

Using your own sleep diary, do all the calculations we've discussed, and fill in your average sleep efficiency for this past week below:

*My current sleep efficiency is:* __ *percent.*

If you're at 85 percent or higher, you might be in pretty good shape in this department. Your sleep may not be perfect, but you're following the sleep science here, and that's great. Your challenge may be to *keep it up*, especially in regard to stimulus control—because it stinks to get up out of bed at night when we can't sleep, this is where a lot of patients start to slip. And if your sleep efficiency is looking good, yet you're still unhappy with your sleep, hang tight—we're going to come back to this topic shortly.

With Gordon, who had a sleep efficiency in the low 60s, it was clear where we had to start: first of all, *stimulus control*. He really needed to be getting up when he wasn't sleepy or falling asleep. But there is a second strategy we worked on together—

one of the fastest and most effective ways to fix sleep efficiency and get people's sleep processes back in line: *sleep restriction.*

## Sleep Restriction: Build Up That Sleep Pressure

Your homeostatic sleep drive is your secret weapon here. What we're going to do is use your sleep data to ramp up your sleep pressure by, basically, holding that balloon closed as it fills and fills to its maximum capacity. This isn't rocket science: We're going to make you tired. Really tired. This is how we teach your body how to sleep again: when to sleep, where to sleep, and how to "let go" into sleep more quickly and easefully.

With Gordon, step one was to change his sleep schedule. We reduced his "sleep opportunity" to exactly the length of time he was *actually* sleeping, plus a half hour. Remember: you can't shut down like a computer . . . not even when your sleep pressure is about to burst your balloon. It always takes a little bit of time to transition, and we build that in. And when we reduce your sleep opportunity down to more precisely match how much you're actually sleeping on a typical night, we are *not* wanting you to wake up earlier. We need you to stay up later. In the clinic, I almost never say to anybody, "I want you to be asleep by ___ time." What I say all the time is, "I don't want you to go to bed *any earlier* than ___." In Gordon's case, the fill-in-the-blank answer there was *1 a.m.*

Sound extreme? Well, yeah, it is. Sleep restriction can be a little extreme. Sometimes when we do this in the lab, we have people stay at the sleep clinic so they can be monitored. We ask them not to drive during the sleep restriction period, or to do anything else that might be dangerous for themselves or others. (If this approach sounds too extreme for you, or if you have a health issue that would make this inadvisable, fear not—when we get to the practice instructions, I'll be offering a gentler, more gradual version of this called *sleep compression*, where you start bumping your bedtime back bit by bit instead.) But here's an important note about this method: for most people who are struggling with sleep, the "sleep restriction" intervention doesn't actually result in them getting *less sleep* than they have been getting. It results simply in *less time in bed*. If we wanted to be exact, we could call it "time in bed restriction," because so often, that's what it is. When I have you do this, I'm not taking away any sleep. We know how much you're sleeping, because we've tracked and calculated it. We're simply *packaging* your sleep—consolidating it, and then shifting it later—to both rev up your homeostatic sleep drive so you can fall asleep and stay asleep, and to decondition you from associating your bed with wakefulness and struggle.

That said, if your sleep efficiency is low, the first few bedtimes of your "time in bed restriction" can be pretty late, when you do the math and figure out what time you're getting in bed tonight. Gordon was startled by the prescription at first. "I have to *stay up* until 1 a.m.?" he cried. It was three hours past when his husband went to bed, and Gordon was an extrovert—highly social, he preferred to spend his leisure time with a companion. He wasn't used to filling that much downtime on his own. I advised him to spend this time in the living room, where he could relax on the couch and watch his shows, read the magazine articles he kept open in the browser on his phone, never finding time during the day to read them, or catch up on friends' Instagram feeds (as long as it stayed relaxing and didn't veer into mindless semi-engaged scrolling or stressful self-comparison—I recommended he set a timer to make sure he didn't get sucked in and lose too much time in there).

"It's not like you're sleeping anyway," I told him. He conceded the point.

Gordon was at the farthest end of the sleep restriction spectrum that we'll go—we never go down past five hours. Even if people are suffering from bad insomnia and their actual time asleep is much less than that, five is the lowest we'll go. Our goal here is to accumulate sleep debt that'll make falling asleep and staying asleep easier, *not* to totally destroy you.

Typically, we begin our sleep-restriction process by shooting for about a week of sticking to this new, late bedtime. Here's what patients experience: their sleep debt begins to accumulate. Now, during their wind-down time, they are super tired. They're watching the clock and waiting for their prescribed bedtime—whether it's 1 a.m., midnight, 11 p.m., or even 10 p.m., it begins to feel like a struggle to stay awake long enough to make it. When they do climb into bed, they report that it takes them ten minutes or less to drop off. Middle-of-the-night wake ups plummet, too: they don't wake up at all, or maybe only once per night. But most importantly, when they *do* wake up, they're often carrying so much extra sleepiness that they're more likely to drop back to sleep.

Before the week was up, Gordon's sleep efficiency had rocketed up to almost 93 percent. He was making it to 1 a.m., falling asleep almost instantly, and not waking up until Ben's alarm chirped at 6:30 a.m. He was sleeping for a solid five and a half hours, but physically in bed for less than six. He was falling asleep quickly and effortlessly, and staying asleep across the night—the only problem was, he wasn't getting *enough* sleep. So we shifted to the next phase of sleep restriction: backing off the late bedtime and widening the sleep opportunity, bit by bit. We go in fifteen minute increments every few days, shifting the falling-asleep time earlier and earlier over a matter of weeks. As long as people are still falling asleep quickly and staying asleep through the night (for the most part), we keep moving the bedtime earlier.

When they start to struggle, we pause there and look closer. Maybe we've hit their ideal sleep window; maybe something else is going on. But through this process, we gradually come to an understanding of what works for them in terms of an ideal sleep schedule. One thing we see frequently with patients in the clinic is that when they first come in with their sleep diary, it turns out that they are giving themselves a sleep-opportunity window that is simply much too wide. People have had to work so hard to fall asleep, and have developed such a conditioned arousal problem, that they're in bed for ten hours, sleeping or trying to sleep. That's way too long.

Gordon started with a reasonable sleep-opportunity window—he was physically in bed for about eight and a half hours. For a lot of people, that works. For Ben, it was great! But

Gordon, though he loves Ben to death, is not Ben. As it turned out, his body just didn't need quite that much sleep. Your body is its own sleep-production system—all of us humans, when healthy, can really only produce so much. But within the "healthy, normal" window, there is a range. Ben was happiest with a solid eight hours of sleep, or maybe even a little more. Gordon maxed out at around seven. And he was naturally a night owl—his circadian rhythm was such that he struggled with an early wake-up time. For Ben and Gordon, the solution was to separate sex or physical intimacy and sleep, and not to keep them in the same bucket. They needed two different bedtimes, and that was fine. They figured out new routines for shared activities, togetherness, and intimacy. And Gordon found that he really enjoyed the alone time at night—it was something that really refreshed and relaxed him, and he hadn't even realized it. After our sleep-restriction experiment, we landed on a bedtime of about 11:30. p.m., give or take a half hour, and it's been working well for him. Most nights he can fall asleep quickly, he feels good during the day, and sleep no longer seems like such a struggle.

## A Tougher Nut to Crack

Remember Myra? We met her a few chapters ago, when we were talking about nighttime rumination and how to beat it. She's the super active, busy, outgoing patient of mine who just couldn't relate to the idea of watching clouds drift across the sky. The "trainspotting" tactic we came up with did help her let go of intrusive thoughts. But Myra had a lot of sleep challenges, and we needed to use everything in our arsenal to help her. It was especially urgent because of her epilepsy situation—her doctors believed that improving her sleep might be the one thing that could save her from another brain resection.

One thing that was happening with Myra is that she had gotten extremely anxious about her sleep. It made sense—there was so much riding on it. In Myra's case, her doctors had told her that it was quite possibly the major key to her health and to avoiding a major, invasive surgery that would take months to recover from. That's a lot of pressure. But even if you don't have the kind of stakes riding on your sleep that Myra did, sleep anxiety is a real thing. We all know how important it is. We know conceptually that in the long term, it's critical for our health and longevity. And we also know how we feel when we don't get enough—we experience firsthand the energy drop, the short temper, the cognitive fuzziness, the lessened ability to enjoy our day. A huge percentage of the patients I see in the clinic, probably 90 percent or so, are struggling with sleep anxiety—it's common and quite widespread. And it's ironic that often the biggest thing standing between ourselves and our sleep is *nervousness* about sleep.

This is where sleep restriction can be super effective: we rev up that homeostatic sleep drive until it overwhelms the anxiety that's getting in your way. We can use your natural, increased sleep pressure to overcome even the most challenging anxieties and beliefs about sleep. In Myra's case, we had some significant challenges. She had developed a whole suite of rituals surrounding going to bed that she'd become dependent on, but they were so highly specific, they were making sleep even harder to achieve. Not only was her sleep suffering, but her life was becoming more and more restricted.

She believed that once she finally got really sleepy at bedtime, if anything disrupted that sleepiness at all, she would no longer be able to fall sleep. A lot of the rituals she'd established had to do with that. Almost every night, she started to fall asleep on the couch, and then her husband carried her to bed—she believed so strongly that if she walked there herself, she'd "wake up too much." Same with lights. All the lights in the bedroom had to be off when they walked in, or she couldn't fall asleep. If she even encountered a bright light on the way to the bedroom, it was the same. They had a Google nest in the hallway, which puts out a gentle glow—even that was enough to wake her up too much to sleep. She'd gotten in the habit of covering it with her hands while she went past. These conditions were just too precise to meet reliably; they set her up for failure if any small thing went "wrong."

I certainly understood where these requirements had come from—the pressure on her to improve her sleep was intense, and these were a type of coping mechanism, an attempt to control conditions so that they were "perfect" for sleep. What she'd lost was any faith in her own body and sleep processes. To her, sleep was so fragile, anything could completely derail it. And worse, she was missing out on stuff. If she was ever away from home, in a new or unfamiliar place, she'd have insurmountable insomnia. One weekend, she headed to a long-anticipated bachelorette party with a group of her closest friends in Palm Springs, a couple of hours away from her home in Los Angeles. It was sup-posed to be a long weekend of bonding and celebration. But the first night there, she couldn't sleep at all. She was awake till dawn. She called her husband the next day to drive out and pick her up; she ended up missing out on this experience that was really important to her because of her insomnia.

This kind of thing is pretty typical with people who suffer from insomnia. They have protective behaviors that actually reinforce the insomnia. They reify the idea that you can only sleep in a specific place, under specific conditions. And then this becomes true.

Myra was desperate to improve her sleep. For one thing, there was the epilepsy issue. She was highly motivated to ame-liorate her illness through sleep improvement instead of major brain surgery. And secondly, she wanted her life back.

So we worked intensively for months to improve her sleep. She was one of the most dedicated, fiercest sleep patients I've had in the lab. She threw herself wholeheartedly into every in-tervention we introduced, and we did the whole suite of things: Stable wake-up time. Get sunlight exposure in the morning. Scheduled worry time and "trainspotting" to deal with the cog-nitive stuff. And critically, *sleep restriction*. We really pared back her time in bed to get to a good sleep efficiency. This was critical in helping her to overcome the rituals she'd developed to deal with her sleep anxiety. When sleep pressure is higher, it's so much easier to let go of the ritual and realize you *can* fall asleep without it.

One of the ways we treat sleep anxiety is to create an "anxiety hierarchy." We make a list of all the worries and rituals surrounding sleep and bedtime, and rank them according to severity. Then we start removing things, starting with the easiest and progressing to the hardest. A few days into her sleep-restriction week, I suggested Myra stop covering up the glowing Google nest on her way to bed.

"Just give it a try," I said. "It's an experiment."

It worked. We progressed to the next sleep ritual, and the next. She was falling asleep more easily because of her increased sleep pressure, sure, but at the same time she was building a sense of sleep skill and mastery. She was realizing that she didn't need any of these rigid conditions in order to sleep—that she *could* produce sleep, all on her own. She was able to relax and let go of a lot of the anxiety she had surrounding bedtime. And by the end, she was going to bed without worrying about lights or other environmental concerns. She was able to fall asleep pretty quickly. Her sleep was really well consolidated—she had an efficiency in the upper 80s. Her seizures had reduced considerably and her epilepsy was well managed—she never did have to have that brain surgery. And I feel pretty confident that the next time she goes on a weekend trip with friends, she'll have a great time.

## There's No Such Thing as Perfect Sleep

Myra will probably always have sleep challenges. The thing about insomnia is that having it in the past is the best predictor of having it in the future. It's always kind of rattling around back there, and can flare up, especially during times of stress or big change. That's to be expected, and it's not a sign of failure or cause for alarm. These interventions we've been working on this week, including sleep restriction, are strategies that people often have to return to when sleep once again, for whatever reason, presents a challenge. They aren't a one-time-fixes-all kind of thing. These "sleep levers" that we've been talking about require adjusting. Our sleep needs change as we age; they change with illness or parenthood, with new jobs and new places. Being flexible and aware of yourself and your body's needs is part of this.

Myra, once she was sleeping well again, ran up against another issue: her new sleep needs were hard for her to adjust to conceptually. As we were doing the sleep-restriction phase of her treatment, she found that she was really just too tired to get through the day and was having to nap. I was concerned about this initially—it does steal away some of that homeostatic sleep drive that we're trying to leverage for an easy time at bedtime. But her reality is that she is still in recovery. The road to health from epilepsy as serious as hers, and a major brain surgery, is long. It's more of a process than she would like. We ended up scheduling her naps—she takes a one-hour nap most days, which is probably longer than would be good for most people, but works perfectly for her. Her sleep is still nicely consolidated, with good efficiency, and she's falling asleep well at night. From a sleep-health perspective, it's working great. The problem became more that she didn't want to be "a napper"—the idea ran contrary to her ideas about what it means to be healthy and productive. Before her illness progressed, she'd been a teacher, a job she loved—interacting with her students was a huge source of energy and fulfillment for her. But teaching is also quite demanding. She's working her way back into the educational system as a teaching assistant, which is great, but she is anxious to be "back to her old self." So for her, part of being able to have healthy restorative sleep is being OK with her current needs, and to reckon with the ways that her self-image of an active, busy, ambitious person don't exactly match up with what her body is telling her it needs right now. She's having to adjust.

She's come an incredible distance though, and I'm so proud of her—she has even been able to drop all of the sleep medications she was using before we began, and by the time she left our care, was gearing up to start a new full-time job in the school system. Sleep restriction is such an effective method: it makes weaning people off sleep medications so much easier, because it replaces the drug with real sleepiness. There are plenty of scenarios where sleep meds are great and advisable, but I see a lot of people who've become dependent on them as the only way to cross over into sleep, and they arrive with the goal of being able to do it on their own, without that pharmaceutical assist. And many of them can—there is no medical reason that they can't. When we systemically reduce sleep opportunity, they're able to practice that, and to gain a sense of mastery. They see that their sleep *works*. If they can just let things unfold the way they're supposed to, it will happen. They cease to have this high level of anxiety, the voice asking, *Will I be able to sleep tonight?* And importantly, they are able to hang on to this confidence even when sleep doesn't go well. They can have a bad night and be OK the next day, knowing that their building sleep pressure is just going to help them recoup and recover. They know now that any one given night isn't all that important.

My oldest son is ten years old and my youngest is five. What that means for me is that I basically haven't slept that well in ten years—I still get woken up constantly in the middle of the night, and while sometimes I can fall right back asleep, other times I'm up, kept awake by worries or stressors that seem to pop right up in the wee hours like a jack-in-the-box. I spend my days studying the impact of sleep on the immune system, on cognition, on stress; I know how critical sleep is. I also know that my own sleep is imperfect, a fluctuating process. Sometimes my job gets in the way and I go against my own advice. Sometimes life gets in the way. There are all kinds of things outside of our control that will interrupt or degrade our sleep. We can never know for sure that we'll sleep well tonight. But if you're putting pressure on yourself, you've already lost the battle. Sleep is variable, and that's OK! When we have a bad night of sleep, we naturally end up compensating later: the next night of sleep is easier and more restorative.

Sleep patterns vary significantly over the course of a life. Teenagers need much more. Older adults may need less, and often have to adjust their lifestyle to compensate for a shorter sleep time than they've been accustomed to. Hormonal changes in perimenopause and menopause, like estrogen levels dropping, can cause sleep disturbances that leave people waking up more frequently and wondering what they can do to combat it. But often, with the patients I see in the clinic, what helps more than anything is a degree of acceptance about the "sleep phase" they're in. Dr. Gladys McGarey, known as the "Mother of Holistic Medicine" and who's been a practicing MD since the 1940s, celebrated her hundredth birthday in 2020. One of her secrets to health and happiness? When she wakes up in the middle of the night—which for her, has happened frequently during many periods of her life—she doesn't worry about it. She works on one of her many projects, or practices her hymns.

Besides, sleeping through the night in one big chunk, it turns out, might not be the norm for humans historically. Sleep researchers are discovering evidence that up until the 1800s, it was much more common for people to have "bi-phasic" sleep, or to sleep in two distinct segments. Literature from that era makes reference to the "first sleep" or "second sleep"; it seems to have been common for people to be up and about for an hour or two in the middle of the night. During that time, people would write letters, read, have sex, or even get up and do chores like sewing or chopping wood. Others reported using the time for daydreaming or quiet contemplation, meditation, rehashing their dreams. Some were quite active, even paying visits to friends. Historian Roger Ekritch, who has extensively researched sleep through the ages, points out that what's notable about these accounts is how normal it all was—these middle-of-the-night activities are referred to quite casually, with the overall sense that it was common or even typical.[1]

In the early 1990s, sleep researcher Thomas Wehr ran an experiment[2] where participants lived for a month in an environment with a "short photoperiod": only ten hours total of light, as would have naturally occurred for preindustrial humans in many parts of the globe. He found that within just a couple of weeks, people's sleep episodes expanded and then divided into two symmetrical segments with a one- to three-hour wake window in between them. The results closely echoed the reports of the "two sleeps" that were apparently typical of the seventeenth and eighteenth centuries. Obviously our world is different now, with electrically and digitally extended days, and we're not going backward in terms of technology. That said, it's worth noting that there's nothing "natural" or biologically predetermined about sleeping for a solid eight hours a night. In fact, that may be more of a recent phenomenon for us humans— we also believe that for prehistoric humans, sleep was often short or interrupted.

Every few years, the idea of the historical "two sleeps" cycles back into the media discourse on sleep and sleep science; pieces on the topic are enthusiastically passed around on social media. I think we find the concept so compelling because it points to a time period when middle of the night wakefulness wasn't considered a problem to be fixed, but simply a reality to live with or even take advantage of. That's not to say that if you're losing lots of sleep at night and feeling exhausted during the day, you should just live with it—not at all. But it may help to know that wee-hours wakefulness is not inherently bad, unusual, or a clinical indication that something is "wrong." If you came into the sleep lab and told me you were waking up in the middle of the night, the only thing I'd ask you is, "Well, how do you feel?" That's what this all comes down to. We're not trying to fit your sleep into one "ideal model"—there isn't one. We're trying to get you to the point where you're getting the restorative rest your brain and body need, and where you feel like you have the resources to meet the challenges of your day. So if you need help in that department, let's try this week's last and most powerful intervention—this time based on your specific sleep data that you've been gathering.

## TODAY'S PRACTICE

# STAY UP LATE!

If a friend complained to you that they were tired, you'd probably advise them to go to bed early. Today, to fix your sleep, we're doing the opposite. We're going to really fire up your homeostatic sleep drive so that you can start falling asleep more easily and build skill and confidence around sleep.

If you filled out the chart earlier in the chapter, then you've already found your sleep efficiency. If you haven't, then flip back and do that now. If your sleep efficiency is lower than 85 percent, this exercise will really help you—I'd highly recommend giving it a real shot, which means sustaining this practice not only tonight, but over the course of the next week. If you stick to it, you can see results in as little as a week.

If your sleep efficiency is good, but you're still feeling like you struggle with falling asleep or staying asleep, you may want to give this a try anyway! We use this tactic with basically everyone who presents with clinical insomnia. But even for those who don't have a clinical diagnosis, compressing your sleep window can really be effective.

For this exercise, you'll need a couple key pieces of information from that chart:

*Average sleep opportunity:* _____

*Average time asleep:* _____

Your goal here is to close this gap. And we're going to do

that by dramatically cutting down your sleep-opportunity window to more closely match your actual time asleep— even if that amount of time isn't actually enough. We'll adjust for that later.

For tonight: take your average total time asleep (even if that sleep is fragmented; just add up all the segments) and add a half hour. That's your sleep opportunity for tonight. To find your bedtime, start with the wake-up time you've been sticking to this week and go backward by that exact amount of time. You should not be getting into bed before then.

*My sleep opportunity tonight is:* _____ *hours*

*My bedtime tonight is:* _____ *p.m. / a.m.*

Remember: we don't go below a sleep-opportunity window of five hours. And use common sense—if you're compressing your sleep window by a lot, you may need to avoid driving or anything that may seem risky when too sleepy. Additionally, do not attempt without the supervision of a clinician if you have a history of seizures or bipolar disorder as these conditions can be exacerbated by sleep deprivation.

If you can, commit to this bedtime and this compressed sleep window for one week. Use the sleep diary to keep track of when you get in bed, when you fall asleep, and when you wake up. If, after a full week of trying this, your numbers are looking good, and most especially, if you're *feeling* the difference (falling asleep quickly, and staying asleep, for the most part), then I'll recommend that you start backing off the compressed sleep window in small increments of fifteen minutes every couple of nights. As you make your bedtime earlier little by little, keep tracking your sleep with your sleep diary. For some, expanding out your window every couple nights is fine, for others it should be done more slowly, adding fifteen minutes every week, for instance.

For tonight and the next six nights, however, *don't* back it off. You're going to start to feel tired. You're going to be watching the clock at night, wanting the time until bedtime to go faster. Good. That means it's working!

### The Gentler Option: Sleep Compression

For some, full-on sleep restriction will be too extreme, especially outside a clinical setting where I can help you set limits and stick to them. That's OK. If sleep restriction is a no-go for you for whatever reason, try this reverse approach: start bumping your bedtime *back*, to more gradually close the gap between your sleep opportunity and your actual sleep. For folks who choose this method, I recommend bumping back by half-hour increments. So if you normally go to bed at 10 p.m., then tonight you'd go to bed at 10:30 p.m., tomorrow at 11 p.m., and so on. You stop and hold at a bedtime when you start falling asleep more easily.

Sleep compression is a slower process because you're not capturing sleep pressure starting on the first night. You don't immediately start building up homeostatic sleep drive. It takes a lot longer, and in the clinic, we have observed that people are more likely to give up on this method before it has the chance to work. They try it out, and then a couple nights in, they say, "This isn't working and I'm tired; I'm just going to go to bed at my usual time." If you try this method, be systematic about it. Give it at least a week. Sleep restriction is much faster—it's like a shock to the system, like pressing a reset button. You may struggle with daytime tiredness a lot more during the restriction period, but you'll also see results faster. If you choose sleep compression, realize that it will have a longer, slower, gentler arc.

## Troubleshooting

### Don't Sleep In!

Sleep restriction hinges on your commitment to our day-one practice: choosing a wake-up time and sticking to it. This can get challenging for people as the week goes on and they start to really feel the impact of that sleep pressure. Weekends are a trip-up spot; couples who have different schedules can also have a bit more trouble. Do what you need to do to adhere to that stable wake time: set multiple alarms; use a really obnoxious song as your alarm ringtone, like blasting "Eye of the Tiger"; have your partner promise to drag you out of bed, kicking and screaming if necessary. Whatever it takes.

### Track Your Data!

Keep up with your sleep diary. With any experiment, you want to be able to compare the numbers. Sleep restriction can be challenging! It will be essential to be able to look at last week compared to this week, to see how this experimental project of drastically cutting down your sleep window is affecting your sleep.

### And If This Just Doesn't Work for You . . .

That's OK. I'd love for you to give this a real shot, since what we see in the clinic is that it really works for most people. Cognitive behavioral therapy for insomnia is effective for the majority of people who are referred to the clinic, and sleep restriction is a key piece of why it works for them. But for a smaller slice of the people we see, the process just isn't effective.

In these cases, we come back to the core goal. Fixing people's sleep, as much as it is important for health, immune system, cognition, and more, is really all about improving their *waking* function. And there are other ways to improve our days. For instance, we can build naps into our days. One of the ways that the "two sleeps" idea persists into the present day is with cultures that practice the siesta, having a culturally sanctioned afternoon break for rest and napping might decrease total sleep time at night, but is also associated with improved cognition and alertness, as well as reduced risk of heart disease. In Japan, a country known for its intense work culture, people practice something called "inemuri," which might look like napping at your desk or on the subway, but which roughly translates to "sleeping while present." There, a quick nap in public isn't viewed as slothful or lazy, but a sign of dedication and hard work.[3]

While our culture might need a little more prodding to get more comfortable with the midday nap, there's nothing inherently wrong about napping, if nights are persistently hard for you and you can work it into your schedule. But this is sometimes a scenario where medications are particularly appropriate and helpful. There's a new class of medications that are particularly effective with what we call "sleep maintenance": falling asleep and *staying asleep*. When people are waking in the middle of the night or early in the wee hours of the morning, it can be really challenging or impossible to get back to sleep—you've already drained out too much sleep pressure and even if you still feel tired, there's just not enough juice left in your homeostatic sleep drive to get you there.

Finally, it's entirely possible that you are just wrong about how much sleep you need. If you look it up on the internet, you're going to find a billion articles recommending that you get a minimum of seven hours. And yes, that's true for most people—most of us do need that much for the dishwasher of the brain to flush out all the junk, refresh and restore us, and keep us in fighting shape. But there are also people who are genetically "short sleepers."[4] They are simply able to do all that more efficiently, in less time. One guy who came into the sleep clinic fell into this category—he was waking up early in the morning because his body simply would not "make" that much sleep. And he didn't need it. He felt fine, and he was in good health. In the end, it turned out that he just needed to feel OK about sleeping less.

An important caveat: don't use this as an excuse to scrimp on sleep! Statistically speaking, you are probably *not* genetically a short sleeper. This all comes down to how you feel. If you feel good, quite possibly you are good.

### Embrace Imperfect Sleep

If you're awake, and nothing's working, try acceptance. Trust your body: you'll make up for it tomorrow. Remember that any sleep debt you build up, you can use to help yourself fall asleep with more ease the next night. You have this awake time now, in the middle of the night—that's not your choice, but you can choose what to do with it. So do something that makes you happy; something you don't always have time for during a typical busy day. This is "bonus time." Read a book. Watch reruns of *Friends* or *The Real Housewives of Whatever*—nobody's judging. And remember that even the "best" sleepers have bad nights: perfection is not the goal, nor is it possible. Your nights, like your days, will always have a degree of unpredictability. Part of the project of improving our sleep is being OK with that, and knowing that our bodies are resilient and will recover—if we continue to prioritize sleep, realize its value, and live our days according to that knowledge.

# RENEWING YOUR PRESCRIPTION

## THIS IS THE BEGINNING, NOT THE END

JUNE IS IN HER SEVENTIES. SHE LIVES ALONE IN A SUNNY LITTLE DU-plex in Oakland filled with plants, and takes the bus into San Francisco to the sleep clinic to see us. She works at a local nonprofit and regularly volunteers—she's very busy and active in her community, and has no plans to retire any time soon. During the pandemic, she finally let her hair go gray—the slow fade from the coppery bronze she used to dye it, to a bright silky silver, was a way of marking pandemic time. She said she liked her silver hair and was happy for an excuse to finally stop buying boxes of dye. She doesn't mind getting older—"It's better than the alternative!" is what she always says.

What she does mind is that she can't sleep. And she hasn't been able to for most of her life.

Her insomnia started when she was a teenager. Falling asleep became more and more of a struggle. She'd wake up in the middle of the night, too, for no reason she could discern, and then would lie there awake in the dark, unable to drift back off. This has been going on for decades now. Sometimes it's a little better, other times worse, but there seems to be no real rhyme or reason to it. One thing she has noticed is that as she has bad night of sleep after bad night of sleep, she'll get more and more exhausted, until finally she crashes and has a kind of sleep-pressure rebound where she sleeps normally for a couple of nights. And it feels great! But then that sleep pressure wears off, and she's back to her chronic insomnia.

The worst part about it all, she says, is the unpredictability. She never knows what tonight will bring, and this unpredictability fills her day with angst about the coming night.

When her sleep is poor, which is often, she feels bad during the day, too. She's sluggish and irritable. She feels cognitively foggy. She worries that her sleep deficit is causing memory problems, exacerbating the typical issues of aging. By the time she appeared in the clinic, referred by her physician, she was basically resigned to being an insomniac forever. And frankly, I didn't blame her! When I asked her questions about her sleep habits and the patterns of her days, she was doing so many things right. She didn't drink at all—as a recovering alcoholic, it had been decades since she'd had so much as a sip. She wasn't a coffee or soda drinker, so no caffeine. She got a lot of exercise. She didn't think it was possible to change her sleep. And she was a bit apprehensive about even trying. Her question was: "Am I just doomed to be chasing something that's just out of reach?"

Embracing *imperfect* sleep is one thing. It's a big part of washing away sleep anxiety and being OK, confident, happy, and functional when things don't go exactly as planned—which is, let's face it, much of life! But I don't want you to come away from this book believing that you just need to accept poor sleep and live with it. If you feel bad, and your sleep is bad, then let's take action to fix it. To basically every person who's ever walked into my sleep clinic, I've said, "We can make your sleep better." And we do.

With June, we did everything—all the steps you've just done this week, but for even longer, hammering these new habits in over the course of months. She was game for it all, even though she doubted any of it would work. She had no trouble shifting to a consistent wake-up time, or nudging bedtime back to improve her sleep efficiency—the idea of the "sleep pressure balloon," and intentionally filling it up, really made sense to her. We had some tussles over the stimulus control, though—she was really attached to her bedtime routine, which involved doing sudoku on her iPad and listening to podcasts, in bed. It didn't take too much effort to convince her to switch away from podcasts like Radio Lab—she got caught up in the stories ("Oh yeah, I've always wanted to learn about Poland's Independence Day!) so it perpetuated not sleeping, since she wanted to listen to the end. The puzzle habit was a harder one to break. She truly believed she had to do the sudoku puzzles *in bed*—she'd do it until she felt sleepy, then toss the iPad aside and close her eyes. She was using it as a sleep aid.

I pushed her to do it outside of bed—I wanted her to experience the transition of falling asleep. In the end, we met in the middle: she had pretty significant arthritis pain that made it uncomfortable for her to move around at night, so I said, "OK, do your puzzles in bed. But sit up, on the opposite side of the bed from where you sleep, and play some ocean waves or music or something—*not* a podcast."

She grudgingly agreed.

In our last meeting, she expressed utter shock that things had actually turned around for her on the sleep front.

"How could I go fifty years, and then happen upon these simple changes . . . and it *works*?" she said. "I never thought this was possible."

Her sleep isn't perfect now, but it's a whole heck of a lot better. The main thing is: *it's predictable*. She can see the consistency and the progress. Some nights are better than others, but sleep is now something she can count on for the first time in her life. She's confident that she can get enough regular sleep that she can do what she really wants to with her life and feel pretty good. And when she does wake up in the middle of the night, she's less pessimistic. She has some agency—it no longer feels like things are just happening *to* her. She appreciates that her sleep is not going to be perfect. But she has a level of sleep mastery now that allows her to be—on the whole—both better rested *and* more relaxed about her sleep.

This book has had two major messages. One is that we need to realize how essential sleep is to our well-being—that it's this magical natural medicine that unlocks our capacity to be our best selves, at work, and in relationships, everywhere—and prioritize it, *really* prioritize it, by making space for wind downs, stress-relief practices, and just protecting our sleep time from the demands of work and a nonstop digital world. The second—

which sounds a bit contradictory to the first—is that we also need to not put so much pressure on sleep. A lot of people we see in the clinic have gone past having a healthy respect for sleep and all it does for them, and have developed cycles of thinking where sleep is much more important than it really is: "If I fix my sleep, everything will improve! My job, my marriage, my life, my skin!" What we see is that thinking this way ends up perpetuating the sleep problem.

The truth? It's a balancing act. Both things are true. Yes, you need to prioritize sleep if you want to thrive and be your best self. You need to protect it. Let yourself have the time and space you need for it. Rearrange your day to make it happen. And at the same time, know that you'll be OK after a bad night or two. If you stick to the program, your body will catch up.

## We All Need Access to Restorative Sleep

June's one of my success stories. It's what I aspire to: that everybody who comes through our clinic ends up saying the stuff she says. Sometimes, though, we have to end treatment when people are still anxious or struggling. And that's often because of factors that are completely out of their control. Not every story is a success story, and that's why we need to remove systemic barriers to sleep.

I worked with one woman who lived in a hotel. The stress of housing insecurity was extreme. Plus, she lived in the Tenderloin in San Francisco, a low-income neighborhood with a lot of homelessness and higher crime. She found it hard to sleep because she felt constantly vigilant and was kept awake by neighborhood noise. We worked with her on some strategies, and I hope they helped at least a little, but I remember that when she was leaving our care, I was still wishing there was more we could do for her.

I also see a lot of people in the clinic who struggle to prioritize their sleep the way they should because of work pressures. It's easy to say, "I know I need to make time for sleep so I can be better tomorrow instead of trying to finish work now," and it's another thing to actually *do* it. We are all steeped in a culture that has long valorized late work, short sleep, tiredness as a badge of honor, and productivity above all else. It's really hard to deprogram from that—especially when you have a to-do list as long as your arm, and because we tend to attach a lot of our identity and self-worth to our careers. When there's something important unfinished, it's tough to stick to the script night after night and set it aside to wind down and get the rest you actually need.

When I first started talking about sleep and health to the general public, my first paper on my research on sleep and vaccine efficacy had just been published. The gist of it was basically that sleep impacts immune function—*a lot*. People who got adequate sleep seemed to mount a better immune response to vaccination. They were more protected. And people wanted to know: What did that actually mean for human health? What was the takeaway?

Here's what I told them: What I hoped was that our research findings would raise the profile of sleep as a key pillar of health, one that stands alongside nutrition and exercise but is often overlooked in our society.

That was a decade ago. Have my hopes come true? Well, I think things have improved. People are much more aware of the fact that sleep is critical for health. The value of sleep, in the zeitgeist, has shifted for the better. But it hasn't quite trickled down at a policy level. We're *telling* people that sleep is a critical pillar of health, but we're not necessarily giving them the support, space, and tools to get it. There have been some successes here and there—like movement towards shifting school start times later (to accommodate the real sleep needs of teenagers). But in health care, and in the working world for Western cultures, we're a productivity-driven culture. It's a *time use* model—we seem to want to squeeze every minute out of our workers, without much appreciation for the benefits *to* productivity when people get real rest, or for the health care cost savings that come from protecting the sleep of a population.

So, my question for you, at the end of this week of working on your own sleep, is: do you have any power to influence this for others?

We don't always realize that *we* are the changemakers. That we have influence within the workplace and the culture. That we can help shift norms and expectations. Even improving this for a small group of people—maybe even for *one person*—is significant. What can you do within your sphere? Be a sleep advocate! In your workplace, at your school or your child's school, in your home. Over time, small cultural shifts—just like the small shifts in habit and routine we worked on his week—can have a widening impact. We can change the conversation, change the values we hold as central, change the structures we live inside, change the expectations for all of us. We can build a collective will for change.

## This Is the Beginning, Not the End

I hope you'll think about the long-term cultural project of sleep, which we all play a role in. But what about you? What about tomorrow?

We just finished this week of working on your sleep by making simple yet powerful daily shifts to one aspect of your day or routine. The seven strategies I included here are the ones I know to be the most successful, the most impactful, and the most accessible—you don't need to be in a fancy sleep lab to make these tools work for you.

Let's imagine I'm sending you off from my sleep clinic at UCSF. Here's what I'd say to you as we discharged you, back into your life with your new set of sleep skills:

First: *Keep going!* Don't stop. Let these new habits really become *habits*. For most people, getting to the place where their sleep wasn't working for them anymore didn't happen overnight. It happens over time. Gradually, because of all kinds of factors (jobs, worries, health issues, thought patterns, and more) you build up barriers to sleep. Breaking them down is the same: a process. You have to dismantle those barriers brick by brick, and it can take a little time. I hope you've felt better this week, and that some of these strategies are already working their magic. I hope things feel a little easier already, or at least that you're feeling a bit more in control. But the project of great sleep takes longer than a week. This is the beginning, not the end! And now you have the tools in place to improve your life through improved sleep. Everything we know from the sleep science tells us that for most people, this toolbox of strategies—if we keep doing them consistently, persistently, and patiently—is going to improve both quality and quantity of sleep.

The second thing I say: If you're really having trouble, *don't beat yourself up*. Give it time. We often have to send people off from the clinic still feeling a little anxious about their sleep. If that's the case for you, I don't want you to feel lesser-than, or that you've been unsuccessful. It's perfectly normal. For some of us, the struggle with sleep has become a kind of trauma. It's not adaptive, as a human, to quickly forget about it. That doesn't mean you won't! June changed her sleep after fifty years. It's always possible to improve, no matter your starting point, no matter how long you've been struggling.

The last thing I tell people as they leave my clinic on their last visit: *it's very possible that something's going to happen and your sleep isn't going to be as good as it is now*. Stuff can knock us off our path of sleep improvement. A work or family crisis, or even just the typical pileup of busyness and stress, can set you back. It's easy to feel frustrated when it feels like "one step forward, two steps back." But as your sleep gets better, the more resilient you'll be to the bad nights. A bad night doesn't mean the next night's going to be bad. It probably means the next night's going to be better! "And if it's not, and it gets really bad," I tell my patients, "I'm here."

Within a year after discharge, I'll hear from about 10 percent of my patients who email me with a problem that's cropped up: *XYZ happened and I stopped being able to sleep again! What do I do?*

It's usually typical life stuff: stress management, responsibilities piling up, other things starting to take priority. So here's what I tell them: RESET. Come back to these practices that you *know* work. Life happens—we can't control it—but when it does, you now have a set of strategies to put in place immediately to protect your sleep and get it back on track.

So if you hit a rough patch, come back to this book. Start at day one. Refresh your mind, body, and sleep system with these strategies. Remember what these tools are designed to do: *to get us out of our own way.* Your sleep is always inside you: it's part of who you are as a human. And now you have the tools you need to unlock it.

# ACKNOWLEDGMENTS

It has been an honor to share my passion about sleep through this book. However, none of this would have been possible without an incredible team of professionals. First, I want to express my sincerest gratitude to the whole Idea Architects team, and particularly Rachel Neumann. Rachel, thank you sharing your vision for this book and the entire *Prescription* series. Your commitment to making the world a better place through these books is an inspiration, and I am eternally grateful that you took a chance on me as an author. I look forward to all the good work we will do together in the years to come. I also want to thank all of the other talented people at IA and Penguin Life, including Amy Sun, for shepherding me through the process. I am changed for the better as a result.

This book was only possible because of the incomparable talents of Alyssa Knickerbocker. You are an incredible wordsmith and editor, and your capacity to write is only matched by your wit and humor. I also want to acknowledge the ardent support of my closest colleague at UCSF, Dr. Elissa Epel. You continue to inspire me with your creativity, commitment to rigorous science, and passion to make real-world change.

The stories in this book are fictionalized but based on real conversations with former patients. Their struggles reflect the struggles of so many, and I am grateful for the trust they put in me as a clinician. I am also indebted to my sleep colleagues at UCSF, particularly those who work in our clinic, including Drs. Jennifer Felder, Caterina Mosti, Lauren Asarnow, Liza Ashbrook, and Andrew Krystal. Thank you for your friendship and collaboration in helping our patients get the sleep they sorely need.

There are so many who played such meaningful roles in my development as a researcher, clinician, and person. I would like to express my appreciation to all my mentors and colleagues over the years, especially Drs. Anna Marsland, Steve Manuck, Peter Gianaros, at the University of Pittsburgh, Sheldon Cohen at Carnegie Mellon University, and Nancy Adler at UCSF. I also want to recognize Dr. Martica Hall at the University of Pittsburgh for inspiring me to pursue sleep research in the first place. Tica, thank you for sharing your enthusiasm for the power of sleep with me, it made all the difference. I also want to thank Drs. Jack Edinger and Meg Danforth, who were gracious in training me in cognitive behavioral therapy for insomnia when I was a psychology intern at Duke University Medical Center. I am also grateful to my colleagues who have played such a meaningful role in making my job (and writing this book) so much fun, including Dr. Wendy Berry Mendes, and my weekly writing group made up of Drs. Sarah Pressman, Janet Tomiyama, and Carissa Low. Finally, I want to acknowledge the unwavering support of my family, near and far. I love you all dearly. And to my wife and boys, thank you for putting up with my obsession with sleep all these years. Unfortunately, it will continue.

# APPENDIX 1

## ADDITIONAL RESOURCES

There are lots of different sleep issues that can lead to feeling run-down during the day and not performing at your best. This book was developed to help people with difficulties falling and staying asleep (i.e., insomnia). That means that if you have a different sleep problem, this book may not be the right one for you or at least will not directly address your sleep issue.

Here are a few signs to watch out for that may indicate you have an underlying issue that won't respond to the strategies in this book:

- You're regularly getting seven hours of sleep or more, but still feel tired most days
- You struggle to stay awake while driving or performing other tasks that keep you seated
- You snore loudly, so much so that you can be heard in another room
- You wake up in the middle of the night gasping for breath

- You have an intense, often irresistible, urge to move your legs in the middle of the night
- You suffer from uncontrollable episodes of falling asleep in the daytime, often associated with muscle weakness

If any of the above symptoms sound like you, it would be worth discussing them with your doctor, who may refer you to a sleep specialist.

Finally, if you suffer from insomnia and want more personalized treatment, such as face-to-face (or telehealth) cognitive behavioral therapy for insomnia (CBTI), consider discussing this with your doctor or visit The Society of Behavioral Sleep Medicine at behavioralsleep.org to identify possible providers.

# APPENDIX 2

# YOUR SLEEP DIARY

Hello, and welcome to your sleep diary! The instructions for filling this out are pretty simple. No "*Dear diary*" or deep thoughts required—just the facts, as best as you can estimate them.

Fill this out as soon as you wake up in the morning, each day this week. The best thing to do is keep this book by your bed, with this page bookmarked, so you can flip to it immediately upon awakening. Try to estimate the answers as accurately as you can. As I mentioned in the intro to this sleep diary, I recommend skipping the wearables—they can be inaccurate, over- or underestimate sleep, or even be too specific (we don't actually need to know that you woke up five times for 6.25 minutes . . . maybe you did, but if you didn't remember it, I don't want it on the diary).

Nor do I want you trying to fill this out *while* in the process of falling asleep. You don't want to become hypervigilant about tracking your sleep data, or undermine your falling-asleep process by scrutinizing it so closely. At night, follow the practice instructions in this book and don't worry about being precise. For our purposes, your best guess in the morning is good enough. And when it comes to sleep, we never want the perfect to be the enemy of good-enough.

Note: don't worry about filling in the last three rows (sleep opportunity, time asleep, and sleep efficiency) until you finish reading the day seven chapter. In day seven, I'll explain how to calculate those values. Until then, you can skip those boxes.

Please complete this to the best of your ability.

| Day of the week | | | | | | | |
|---|---|---|---|---|---|---|---|
| Time you tried to fall asleep? | | | | | | | |
| How long it took you to fall asleep (in minutes)? | | | | | | | |
| Number of times you woke up and tried to return to sleep? | | | | | | | |
| How long were you awake during wake times reported above? (Total number of minutes) | | | | | | | |
| Time you woke up for the last time this morning? | | | | | | | |
| What was your sleep quality? (See scale below) | | | | | | | |
| Sleep Opportunity (in minutes) | | | | | | | |
| Time Asleep (in minutes) | | | | | | | |
| Sleep Efficiency | | | | | | | |

**Sleep quality rating scale:** 0 = worst sleep; 25 = poor sleep; 50 = average sleep; 75 = good sleep; 100 = best sleep

*Please complete this to the best of your ability.*

| Day of the week | | | | | | | |
|---|---|---|---|---|---|---|---|
| Time you tried to fall asleep? | | | | | | | |
| How long it took you to fall asleep (in minutes)? | | | | | | | |
| Number of times you woke up and tried to return to sleep? | | | | | | | |
| How long were you awake during wake times reported above? (Total number of minutes) | | | | | | | |
| Time you woke up for the last time this morning? | | | | | | | |
| What was your sleep quality? (See scale below) | | | | | | | |
| Sleep Opportunity (in minutes) | | | | | | | |
| Time Asleep (in minutes) | | | | | | | |
| Sleep Efficiency | | | | | | | |

**Sleep quality rating scale:** 0 = worst sleep; 25 = poor sleep; 50 = average sleep; 75 = good sleep; 100 = best sleep

Please complete this to the best of your ability.

| Day of the week | | | | | | | |
|---|---|---|---|---|---|---|---|
| Time you tried to fall asleep? | | | | | | | |
| How long it took you to fall asleep (in minutes)? | | | | | | | |
| Number of times you woke up and tried to return to sleep? | | | | | | | |
| How long were you awake during wake times reported above? (Total number of minutes) | | | | | | | |
| Time you woke up for the last time this morning? | | | | | | | |
| What was your sleep quality? (See scale below) | | | | | | | |
| Sleep Opportunity (in minutes) | | | | | | | |
| Time Asleep (in minutes) | | | | | | | |
| Sleep Efficiency | | | | | | | |

**Sleep quality rating scale:** 0 = worst sleep; 25 = poor sleep; 50 = average sleep; 75 = good sleep; 100 = best sleep

Please complete this to the best of your ability.

| Day of the week | | | | | | | |
|---|---|---|---|---|---|---|---|
| Time you tried to fall asleep? | | | | | | | |
| How long it took you to fall asleep (in minutes)? | | | | | | | |
| Number of times you woke up and tried to return to sleep? | | | | | | | |
| How long were you awake during wake times reported above? (Total number of minutes) | | | | | | | |
| Time you woke up for the last time this morning? | | | | | | | |
| What was your sleep quality? (See scale below) | | | | | | | |
| Sleep Opportunity (in minutes) | | | | | | | |
| Time Asleep (in minutes) | | | | | | | |
| Sleep Efficiency | | | | | | | |

**Sleep quality rating scale:** 0 = worst sleep; 25 = poor sleep; 50 = average sleep; 75 = good sleep; 100 = best sleep

# NOTES

## INTRODUCTION

1. Aric A. Prather et al., "Sleep and Antibody Response to Hepatitis B Vaccination," *Sleep* 35, no. 8 (August 1, 2012): 1063–69, doi.org/10.5665/sleep.1990.
2. Aric A. Prather et al., "Temporal Links Between Self-Reported Sleep and Antibody Responses to the Influenza Vaccine," *International Journal of Behavioral Medicine*, March 31, 2020, doi.org/10.1007/s12529-020-09879-4; Karine Spiegel, John F. Sheridan, and Eve Van Cauter, "Effect of Sleep Deprivation on Response to Immunization," *JAMA* 288, no. 12 (September 25, 2002): 1471–72, doi.org/10.1001/jama.288.12.1471-a.
3. Aric A. Prather et al., "Behaviorally Assessed Sleep and Susceptibility to the Common Cold," *Sleep* 38, no. 9 (September 1, 2015): 1353–59, doi.org/10.5665/sleep.4968.
4. Adam J. Krause et al., "The Pain of Sleep Loss: A Brain Characterization in Humans," *Journal of Neuroscience: The Official Journal of the Society for Neuroscience* 39, no. 12 (March 20, 2019): 2291–2300, doi.org/10.1523/JNEUROSCI.2408-18.2018.
5. Chandra L. Jackson, Susan Redline, and Karen M. Emmons, "Sleep as a Potential Fundamental Contributor to Disparities in Cardiovascular Health," *Annual Review of Public Health* 36 (March 18, 2015): 417–40, doi.org/10.1146/annurev-publhealth-031914-122838.
6. Luciana Besedovsky, Tanja Lange, and Monika Haack, "The Sleep-Immune Crosstalk in Health and Disease," *Physiological Reviews* 99, no. 3 (March 28, 2019): 1325–80, doi.org/10.1152/physrev.00010.2018.
7. Sirimon Reutrakul, Naresh M. Punjabi, and Eve Van Cauter, "Impact of Sleep and Circadian Disturbances on Glucose Metabolism and Type 2 Diabetes," in *Diabetes in America*, ed. Catherine C. Cowie et al., 3rd ed. (Bethesda, MD: National Institute of Diabetes and Digestive and Kidney Diseases [US], 2018), ncbi.nlm.nih.gov/books/NBK568006/.
8. Veronica Guadagni et al., "The Effects of Sleep Deprivation on Emotional

Empathy," *Journal of Sleep Research* 23, no. 6 (December 2014): 657–63, doi .org/10.1111/jsr.12192; Amie M. Gordon and Serena Chen, "The Role of Sleep in Interpersonal Conflict: Do Sleepless Nights Mean Worse Fights?" *Social Psychological and Personality Science* 5, no. 2 (March 1, 2014): 168–75, doi .org/10.1177/1948550613488952.

9. Mark R. Rosekind et al., "The Cost of Poor Sleep: Workplace Productivity Loss and Associated Costs," *Journal of Occupational and Environmental Medicine* 52, no. 1 (2010): 91–98; Robert Stickgold and Matthew Walker, "To Sleep, Perchance to Gain Creative Insight?" *Trends in Cognitive Sciences* 8, no. 5 (May 2004): 191–92, doi.org/10.1016/j.tics.2004.03.003.

10. Lulu Xie et al., "Sleep Drives Metabolite Clearance from the Adult Brain," *Science* 342, no. 6156 (October 18, 2013): 373–77, doi.org/10.1126/science .1241224.

## BEFORE WE BEGIN

1. Kelly Glazer Baron et al., "Orthosomnia: Are Some Patients Taking the Quantified Self Too Far?" *Journal of Clinical Sleep Medicine: Official Publication of the American Academy of Sleep Medicine* 13, no. 2 (February 15, 2017): 351–54, doi.org/10.5664/jcsm.6472.

## DAY 1: SET YOUR (INTERNAL) CLOCK

1. Nathaniel F. Watson et al., "Recommended Amount of Sleep for a Healthy Adult: A Joint Consensus Statement of the American Academy of Sleep Medicine and Sleep Research Society," *Sleep* 38, no. 6 (June 1, 2015): 843–44, doi.org/10.5665/sleep.4716.

2. Ellen R. Stothard et al., "Circadian Entrainment to the Natural Light-Dark Cycle Across Seasons and the Weekend," *Current Biology* 27, no. 4 (February 20, 2017): 508–13, doi.org/10.1016/j.cub.2016.12.041.

3. Till Roenneberg and Martha Merrow, "The Circadian Clock and Human Health," *Current Biology* 26, no. 10 (May 23, 2016): R432–43, doi.org/10.1016 /j.cub.2016.04.011.

4. Jiu-Chiuan Chen et al., "Sleep Duration, Cognitive Decline, and Dementia Risk in Older Women," *Alzheimer's & Dementia* 12, no. 1 (January 1, 2016): 21–33, doi.org/10.1016/j.jalz.2015.03.004; Francesco P. Cappuccio et al., "Sleep Duration Predicts Cardiovascular Outcomes: A Systematic Review and Meta-Analysis of Prospective Studies," *European Heart Journal* 32, no. 12 (June 1, 2011): 1484–92, doi.org/10.1093/eurheartj/ehr007; Long Zhai,

Hua Zhang, and Dongfeng Zhang, "Sleep Duration and Depression Among Adults: A Meta-Analysis of Prospective Studies," *Depression and Anxiety* 32, no. 9 (2015): 664–70, doi.org/10.1002/da.22386; Yili Wu, Long Zhai, and Dongfeng Zhang, "Sleep Duration and Obesity Among Adults: A Meta-Analysis of Prospective Studies," *Sleep Medicine* 15, no. 12 (December 1, 2014): 1456–62, doi.org/10.1016/j.sleep.2014.07.018.

5. Harald Schrader, Gunnar Bovim, and Trond Sand, "The Prevalence of Delayed and Advanced Sleep Phase Syndromes," *Journal of Sleep Research* 2, no. 1 (1993): 51–55, doi.org/10.1111/j.1365-2869.1993.tb00061.x.

6. Michael Gradisar and Stephanie J. Crowley, "Delayed Sleep Phase Disorder in Youth," *Current Opinion in Psychiatry* 26, no. 6 (November 2013): 580–85, doi.org/10.1097/YCO.0b013e328365a1d4.

## DAY 2: EASE OFF THE GAS

1. Soomi Lee et al., "Daily Antecedents and Consequences of Nightly Sleep," *Journal of Sleep Research* 26, no. 4 (August 2017): 498–509, doi.org/10.1111/jsr.12488.

2. Yang Yap et al., "Bi-Directional Relations between Stress and Self-Reported and Actigraphy-Assessed Sleep: A Daily Intensive Longitudinal Study," *Sleep* 43, no. 3 (March 12, 2020): zsz250, doi.org/10.1093/sleep/zsz250.

3. Jared D. Minkel et al., "Sleep Deprivation and Stressors: Evidence for Elevated Negative Affect in Response to Mild Stressors When Sleep Deprived," *Emotion* 12, no. 5 (October 2012): 1015–20, doi.org/10.1037/a0026871.

4. Amie M. Gordon and Serena Chen, "The Role of Sleep in Interpersonal Conflicts: Do Sleepless Nights Mean Worse Fights?" *Social Psychology and Personality Science* 5, no. 2 (March 1, 2014): 168–75, doi.org/10.1177/1948550613488952.

5. Stephanie M. Greer, Andrea N. Goldstein, and Matthew P. Walker, "The Impact of Sleep Deprivation on Food Desire in the Human Brain," *Nature Communications* 4 (2013): 2259, doi.org/10.1038/ncomms3259.

6. Shantha M. W. Rajaratnam et al., "Sleep Disorders, Health, and Safety in Police Officers," *JAMA* 306, no. 23 (December 21, 2011): 2567–78, doi.org/10.1001/jama.2011.1851.

7. Kyoungmin Cho, Christopher M. Barnes, and Cristiano L. Guanara, "Sleepy Punishers Are Harsh Punishers," *Psychological Science* 28, no. 2 (February 2017): 242–47, doi.org/10.1177/0956797616678437.

8. Christopher M. Barnes et al., "'You Wouldn't Like Me When I'm Sleepy': Leaders' Sleep, Daily Abusive Supervision, and Work Unit Engagement,"

*Academy of Management Journal* 58, no. 5 (October 1, 2015): 1419–37, doi
.org/10.5465/amj.2013.1063.

9. Tanja C. Adam and Elissa S. Epel, "Stress, Eating and the Reward System,"
*Physiology & Behavior* 91, no. 4 (July 24, 2007): 449–58, doi.org/10.1016
/j.physbeh.2007.04.011.

10. Marie-Pierre St-Onge et al., "Fiber and Saturated Fat Are Associated with
Sleep Arousals and Slow Wave Sleep," *Journal of Clinical Sleep Medicine:
Official Publication of the American Academy of Sleep Medicine* 12, no. 1
(2016): 19–24, doi.org/10.5664/jcsm.5384.

11. St-Onge et al., "Fiber and Saturated Fat Are Associated with Sleep Arousals
and Slow Wave Sleep."

12. Elissa S. Epel and Aric A. Prather, "Stress, Telomeres, and Psychopathology:
Toward a Deeper Understanding of a Triad of Early Aging," *Annual Review
of Clinical Psychology* 14 (May 7, 2018): 371–97, doi.org/10.1146/annurev
-clinpsy-032816-045054.

13. Marta Jackowska et al., "Short Sleep Duration Is Associated with Shorter
Telomere Length in Healthy Men: Findings from the Whitehall II Cohort
Study," *PloS One* 7, no. 10 (2012): e47292, doi.org/10.1371/journal.pone
.0047292.

14. Prashant Kaul et al., "Meditation Acutely Improves Psychomotor Vigilance,
and May Decrease Sleep Need," *Behavioral and Brain Functions* 6 (July 29,
2010): 47, doi.org/10.1186/1744-9081-6-47.

## DAY 3: ENERGIZE—BUT DO IT RIGHT

1. Diane C. Mitchell et al., "Beverage Caffeine Intakes in the U.S.," *Food and
Chemical Toxicology: An International Journal Published for the British In-
dustrial Biological Research Association* 63 (2014): 136–42. doi.org/10.1016
/j.fct.2013.10.042.

2. Based on the assumption that each 60kg bag produces around 8,520 cups of
coffee.

3. Marjo H. Eskelinen and Miia Kivipelto, "Caffeine as a Protective Factor in
Dementia and Alzheimer's Disease," *Journal of Alzheimer's Disease* 20,
suppl. 1 (2010): S167–74, doi.org/10.3233/JAD-2010-1404; Laura M. Stevens
et al., "Association Between Coffee Intake and Incident Heart Failure Risk,"
*Circulation: Heart Failure* 14, no. 2 (February 1, 2021): e006799, doi.org
/10.1161/CIRCHEARTFAILURE.119.006799; Rob M. van Dam and Frank B.
Hu, "Coffee Consumption and Risk of Type 2 Diabetes: A Systematic Review," *JAMA* 294, no. 1 (July 6, 2005): 97–104, doi.org/10.1001/jama.294.1.97.

4. Garrett C. Hisler and Jean M. Twenge, "Sleep Characteristics of U.S. Adults Before and During the COVID-19 Pandemic," *Social Science & Medicine* 276 (May 1, 2021): 113849, doi.org/10.1016/j.socscimed.2021.113849; Charles M. Morin et al., "Sleep and Circadian Rhythm in Response to the COVID-19 Pandemic," *Canadian Journal of Public Health* 111, no. 5 (October 1, 2020): 654–57, doi.org/10.17269/s41997-020-00382-7; Rebecca Robbins et al., "Estimated Sleep Duration Before and During the COVID-19 Pandemic in Major Metropolitan Areas on Different Continents: Observational Study of Smartphone App Data," *Journal of Medical Internet Research* 23, no. 2 (February 2, 2021): e20546, doi.org/10.2196/20546.

5. "Effects of Caffeine and Acute Aerobic Exercise on Working Memory and Caffeine Withdrawal | Scientific Reports," accessed February 3, 2022, www.nature.com/articles/s41598-019-56251-y.

6. Elissa S. Epel, "The Geroscience Agenda: Toxic Stress, Hormetic Stress, and the Rate of Aging," *Ageing Research Reviews* 63 (November 2020): 101167, doi.org/10.1016/j.arr.2020.101167.

## DAY 4: WORRY EARLY

1. Amie M. Gordon et al., "Bidirectional Links Between Social Rejection and Sleep," *Psychosomatic Medicine* 81, no. 8 (2019): 739–48, doi.org/10.1097/PSY.0000000000000669.

2. Ethan Kross et al., "Social Rejection Shares Somatosensory Representations with Physical Pain," *Proceedings of the National Academy of Sciences* 108, no. 15 (April 2011) 6270–75; doi.org/10.1073/pnas.1102693108.

3. G. W. Brown and T. O. Harris, *Social Origins of Depression: A Study of Psychiatric Disorder in Women* (New York: Free Press, 1978); Constance Hammen, "Stress and Depression," *Annual Review of Clinical Psychology* 1 (2005): 293–319, doi.org/10.1146/annurev.clinpsy.1.102803.143938.

4. Sally S. Dickerson and Margaret E. Kemeny, "Acute Stressors and Cortisol Responses: A Theoretical Integration and Synthesis of Laboratory Research," *Psychological Bulletin* 130, no. 3 (May 2004): 355–91, doi.org/10.1037/0033-2909.130.3.355; Sally S. Dickerson, Tara L. Gruenewald, and Margaret E. Kemeny, "When the Social Self Is Threatened: Shame, Physiology, and Health," *Journal of Personality* 72, no. 6 (December 2004): 1191–1216, doi.org/10.1111/j.1467-6494.2004.00295.x.

5. Gordon et al., "Bidirectional Links Between Social Rejection and Sleep."

6. Sofia Pappa et al., "Prevalence of Depression, Anxiety, and Insomnia Among Healthcare Workers During the COVID-19 Pandemic: A Systematic Review

and Meta-Analysis," *Brain, Behavior, and Immunity* 88 (August 2020): 901–907, doi.org/10.1016/j.bbi.2020.05.026.

7. "Covid-19: Tracking the Impact on Media Consumption," Nielsen, June 16, 2020, www.nielsen.com/us/en/insights/article/2020/covid-19-tracking-the -impact-on-media-consumption/.

8. Michelle J. Sternthal, Natalie Slopen, and David R. Williams, "Racial Disparities in Health: How Much Does Stress Really Matter?" *Du Bois Review: Social Science Research on Race* 8, no. 1 (2011): 95–113, doi.org/10.1017 /S1742058X11000087.

9. Amie M. Gordon et al., "Anticipated and Experienced Ethnic/Racial Discrimination and Sleep: A Longitudinal Study," *Personality & Social Psychology Bulletin* 46, no. 12 (December 2020): 1724–35, doi.org/10.1177/0146167220 928859.

## DAY 5: YOU ARE NOT A COMPUTER, YOU CAN'T JUST SHUT DOWN

1. Rishi Sharma, Pradeep Sahota, and Mahesh M. Thakkar, "Melatonin Promotes Sleep in Mice by Inhibiting Orexin Neurons in the Periformical Lateral Hypothalamus," *J Pineal Res*, 2018; 65:e12498. doi.org/10.1111/jpi.12498.

2. Anne-Marie Chang et al., "Evening Use of Light-Emitting EReaders Negatively Affects Sleep, Circadian Timing, and Next-Morning Alertness," *Proceedings of the National Academy of Sciences* 112, no. 4 (January 27, 2015): 1232–37, doi.org/10.1073/pnas.1418490112.

3. Chiranth Bhagavan et al., "Cannabinoids in the Treatment of Insomnia Disorder: A Systematic Review and Meta-Analysis," *CNS Drugs* 34, no. 12 (December 2020): 1217–28, doi.org/10.1007/s40263-020-00773-x.

4. Adrian F. Ward et al., "Brain Drain: The Mere Presence of One's Own Smartphone Reduces Available Cognitive Capacity," *Journal of the Association for Consumer Research* 2, no. 2 (April 1, 2017): 140–54, doi.org/10.1086/691462.

5. Dar Meshi, Diana I. Tamir, and Hauke R. Heekeren, "The Emerging Neuroscience of Social Media," *Trends in Cognitive Sciences* 19, no. 12 (December 1, 2015): 771–82, doi.org/10.1016/j.tics.2015.09.004.

6. Joao M. Castaldelli-Maia, Luis E. Segura, and Silvia S. Martins, "The Concerning Increasing Trend of Alcohol Beverage Sales in the U.S. During the COVID-19 Pandemic," *Alcohol* 96 (2021): 37–42, doi.org/10.1016/j.alcohol .2021.06.004.

7. Rachel R. Markwald et al., "Impact of Insufficient Sleep on Total Daily Energy Expenditure, Food Intake, and Weight Gain," *Proceedings of the Na-*

*tional Academy of Sciences* 110, no. 14 (April 2, 2013): 5695–5700, doi.org /10.1073/pnas.1216951110; Yili Wu, Long Zhai, and Dongfeng Zhang, "Sleep Duration and Obesity Among Adults: A Meta-Analysis of Prospective Studies," *Sleep Medicine* 15, no. 12 (December 1, 2014): 1456–62, doi.org/10.1016 /j.sleep.2014.07.018.

8. Christopher M. Barnes et al., "'You Wouldn't Like Me When I'm Sleepy': Leaders' Sleep, Daily Abusive Supervision, and Work Unit Engagement," *Academy of Management Journal* 58, no. 5 (October 1, 2015): 1419–37, doi .org/10.5465/amj.2013.1063; Christopher M. Barnes et al., "Too Tired to Inspire or Be Inspired: Sleep Deprivation and Charismatic Leadership," *Journal of Applied Psychology* 101, no. 8 (August 2016): 1191–99, doi.org/10.1037 /apl0000123.

## DAY 6: (RE)TRAIN YOUR BRAIN

1. I. P. Pavlov, "New Researches on Conditioned Reflexes," *Science* 58, no. 1506 (1923): 359–61, doi.org/10.1126/science.58.1506.359.

## DAY 7: STAY UP LATE

1. A. Roger Ekirch, "Sleep We Have Lost: Pre-industrial Slumber in the British Isles," *American Historical Review* 106, no. 2 (April 2001): 343–86, doi.org /10.1086/ahr/106.2.343.

2. Thomas Wehr, "In Short Photoperiods, Human Sleep Is Biphasic," *Journal of Sleep Research* 1, no. 2 (1992): 103–107, doi.org/10.1111/j.1365-2869.1992 .tb00019.x.

3. Bryant Rousseau, "Napping in Public? In Japan, That's a Sign of Diligence," *New York Times*, December 16, 2006.

4. Guangsen Shi et al., "Mutations in Metabotropic Glutamate Receptor 1 Contribute to Natural Short Sleep Trait," *Current Biology* 31, no. 1 (January 11, 2021): 13–24.e4, doi.org/10.1016/j.cub.2020.09.071.

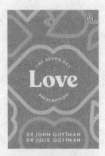
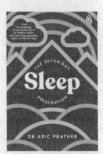
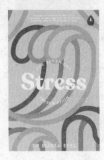